The Gurus' Guide to Serenity

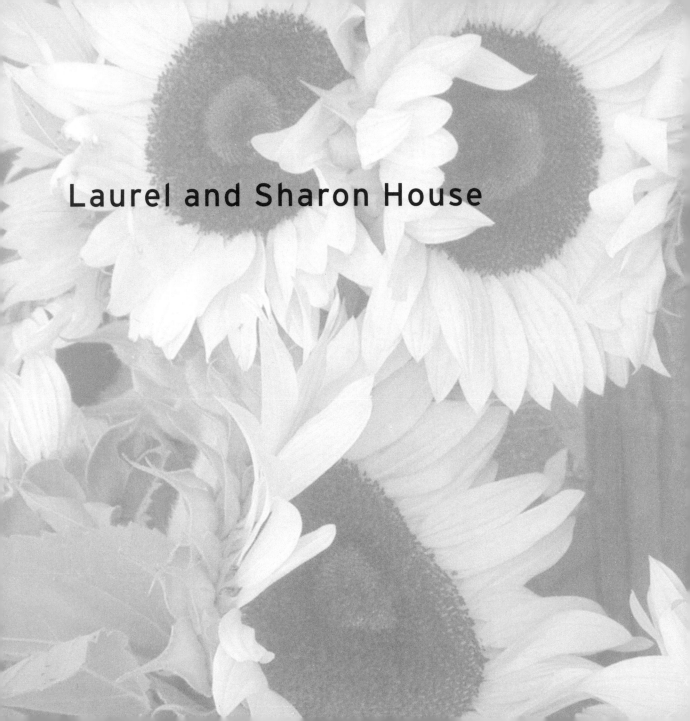

Laurel and Sharon House

The Gurus' Guide to Serenity

A Me-Time Menu of
Celebrity Stress Reducers

wm

WILLIAM MORROW
An Imprint of HarperCollins*Publishers*

HarperCollins books may be purchased for educational, business, or sales promotional use. For information please write: Special Markets Department, HarperCollins Publishers Inc., 10 East 53rd Street, New York, NY 10022.

FIRST EDITION

Designed by Katy Riegel

Printed on acid-free paper

Library of Congress Cataloging-in-Publication Data

House, Laurel.
   The gurus' guide to serenity: a me-time menu of celebrity stress reducers / Laurel and Sharon House.—1st ed.
      p. cm.
    ISBN 0-06-057237-X (alk. paper)
    1. Stress management for women.   2. Relaxation.   3. Celebrities—Health and hygiene. I. House, Sharon (Sharon Wilkinson)   II. Title.

RA785.H678   2004
613'.0424—dc22   2004042488

04   05   06   07   08 ❖/RRD 10 9 8 7 6 5 4 3 2 1

Definition of Guru:

Gu (darkness)
Ru (light)

A guru is one who has the information and knowledge to take one from darkness to light.

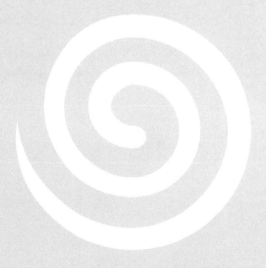

Contents

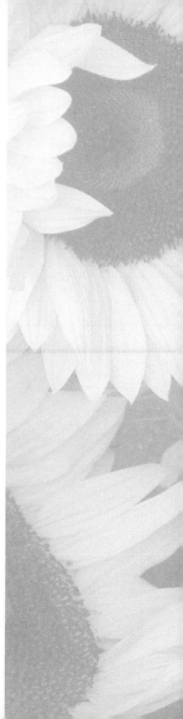

Acknowledgments   xix

Chapter One

Savor Your "Me-Time"   1

Chapter Two

Beauty and the Bath   5

Blissful Baths: The Powerful Potion of Water   5

Tag Galyean's Perfectly Designed Bath   7

Susan Lucci's "Bring Me Back" Baths   11

Garcelle Beauvais-Nilon's Bathroom Sanctuary   12

Lisa Rinna's Bathtub Built for Four   13

Teatime in the Tub   14

Soothing Foot Soaks   16

Chapter Three

Your At-Home Spa   18

Facials, Body Scrubs, and Other Beauty Treatments   18

Glow—Where the "Upper Crust" Go   19

Amber Valletta's Beauty Secrets   27

Arcona Unveils Inner Radiance   28

Garcelle Beauvais-Nilon's Favorite Facial   31

Even Fitness Experts Find Time for Their Faces   32

A Soothing Steam   33

Tracee Ross's Favorite Beauty Secret   35

Healing Spa Water   36

Susan Lucci's Quenching Healthy Habit   38

Chapter Four

Massage . . . The Need to Knead   40

Good Ol' Rubdown   41

Lauren Holly's "Me-Time" Luxury   41

Michelle Kluck's Magic Fingers   42

The Healing Foot Rub   45

Stress Reduction Brow Massage   50

Stressful Jaw Breakers   51

Chapter Five

Finding Your Bliss Through Yoga   53

Total Fitness for Your Body and Mind
   at Kundalini Yoga East   55

Kelly Rutherford's Girl Time   58

Alicia Leigh Willis Cleanses and Energizes   59

Power Yoga to Quiet the Mind   60

Mahshid Tarazi's Sumo to Stretching   62

Janet Gunn Rids the Chatter   63

Anna Getty's Yogic Awakening   64

Chapter Six

Meditation—Relax and Say "Om" 66

Basic Meditation Techniques   69

Jamie Lee Curtis's Meditation Teacher   73

Catherine Hicks on Rosary Beads and Prayer   76

Amber Valletta's Morning and Night Ritual   76

The Art of Being Still   77

Goldie Hawn's Meditation Atrium   81

Shannon Elizabeth's Grounding Meditation   82

Marla Maples's Kabbalah Meditations   83

Chapter Seven

Joyful Cooking   86

Dr. James Rouse on Healing Through Food   88

Dr. James's List of Stress-Management Foods   89

An Afternoon at a Farmers' Market   92

Conscious Cooking with Cary Neff   98

Catherine Hicks on Cooking   112

Akasha's Fabulous Fare   116

Anna Getty's Food Gatherings   117

Chef Elisa Gross's Nurture

    Through Nourishment   119

Marla Maples—One Less Stressed Actress   120

Jenna von Oy's Comforting Cooking 121

Tracee Ross Is "Queen of the Salad" 125

Liquid Yoga 126

Chapter Eight

You've Gotta Have Art 129

Ed and Linda Buttwinick's Safe Haven Art Studio 130

Jane Seymour's Stress-Releasing Refuge 131

Art on the Go 131

Lauren Holly's Artistic Addiction 133

Jenna von Oy's Room Devoted to Crafts 134

Nicole Ritchie's Artistic Antics 135

Asha Blake's Artist Break from Journalism 136

Janet Gunn's Homemade Jewels 139

Grown-up Art Parties 141

Chapter Nine

Nurturing Nature 145

Christie Brinkley's Spirit Replenished 146

Amber Valletta's Weekend Weeding 147

Art Luna's Garden Salon 148

Katherine Whiteside, the "Garden Goddess" 150

Joie Cosentino's Healing Gardens 152

Mark Giebel's Garden 153

A Sanctuary Garden 156

Chapter Ten

Knit One, Purl Too 158

Edith Eig Arouses Impassioned Knitting 158

Justine Bateman Designs 159

Knitting as Therapy 160

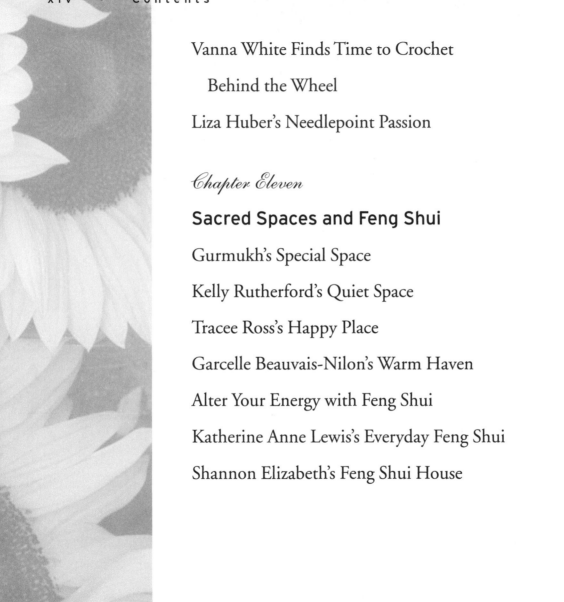

Vanna White Finds Time to Crochet
Behind the Wheel   166

Liza Huber's Needlepoint Passion   168

Chapter Eleven

Sacred Spaces and Feng Shui   169

Gurmukh's Special Space   170

Kelly Rutherford's Quiet Space   173

Tracee Ross's Happy Place   173

Garcelle Beauvais-Nilon's Warm Haven   174

Alter Your Energy with Feng Shui   175

Katherine Anne Lewis's Everyday Feng Shui   178

Shannon Elizabeth's Feng Shui House   184

Chapter Twelve

Work Out Your Body, Work Out Your Mind   188

Dance Your Stress Away   189

Melissa Rivers Relaxes with Her Baby   191

Carnie Wilson and Cardio Barre   191

Cardio Kitchen   193

Kathy Kaehler's Celebrity Circuit Walk   195

Alfre Woodard's Fitness Walk   198

Alicia Leigh Willis Punches Out Her Frustrations   200

Gunnar Peterson's Life-Altering Exercise   200

Amber Valleta's Tension Tamer   203

Mari Winsor's Pilates   204

Susan Lucci's At-Home Exercise Routine   205

Holistic Fitness   206

"Spice Girl" Mel C Finds Her Identity Through Fitness   209

Chapter Thirteen

Little Luxuries 211

Hair Conditioner 212

Amber Valletta's Personal Pleasures 213

Kelly Rutherford Unboggles Her Mind 214

Melissa Rivers Carves Out "Me-Time" 214

Tracee Ross Flips 215

Lauren Holly Breathes 215

Garcelle Beauvais-Nilon Spritzes 216

Susan Lucci Likes Warm Lemon Water 216

Liza Huber's Mindless Moments 217

Chapter Fourteen

Motivation Mantras 218

Setting an Intention 219

Self-Monitoring   220

With a Little Help from a Friend   223

A Gift of Motivation   225

Inner Inspiration   225

The Gift of Giving   226

A Family Affair   226

To Your Health   229

About the Authors   231

Acknowledgments

I would like to thank all of the gurus who have inspired me and my family, and the friends who guide me. Thank you to my husband, Andy, who has always encouraged me; my mother, Beverly, who is a role model; my daughters, Laurel and Julia, who are constantly teaching me; my son, Garth, who loves me unconditionally; my sister, Wendy, who has proven that you can do it all; Elvira for being a rock; Jane and Wendy D for their support; Elizabeth for her enthusiasm; and Linda, who is all I could ever ask for in a friend. —SHARON

What began as a fun idea, floating within one of my many stacks of "idea" files, suddenly turned into a hard-and-fast reality thanks to my mom. Watching myself, in essence, become her prompted this idea in the first place. Then one day she called and said, "Hey, I have this agent coming to town tomorrow (that would be Matthew Guma, our amazing agent). Why don't you jot down that destressing idea of yours and see if he has any interest in developing it into a book?" Suddenly, it was like a whirlwind. Matthew loved the idea, I furnished a proposal, we flew to New York, HarperCollins wanted first dibs, and suddenly my mom and I had a book deal! Thank you, Mom, for your inspiration, inexhaustible friendship, and constant support. Dad, you have always been my role model. Your pride in me makes me constantly strive to do better and achieve more. Elvira, usted es como mi segunda mamá. Gracias por darme su amor incondiciona. Grandpa Bill, I hope I've made you proud. I undoubtedly have a little, okay maybe a lot, of your eccentric, go-getter, spirited personality. Thank you, Julia, for helping me brainstorm ideas and see a fresh perspective. Garth, I know I can count on you no matter what. Thank you for your love. Jagat, thank you for your wisdom, constantly brightening my spirits and encouraging my potential. Rita, I simply would not be here today if it weren't for you. Thank you for taking such an enormous leap of faith with me. To all of my friends who laughed when I told you that I was writing a book on destressing, thank you for forcing me to look at myself and actually practice what I preach. Sometimes people write books on things that they need the most. To our gurus and celebrities, thank you for revealing information about your personal moments. There wouldn't be a *Gurus' Guide* without you. And finally, to my husband, Chris. You are my rock, my sanity, and my balance. Thank you for your love, support, patience, strength, and dedication (not to mention the countless hours you spent editing all of my work). I would not have found this writer within me had it not been for you. I love you.   —LAUREL

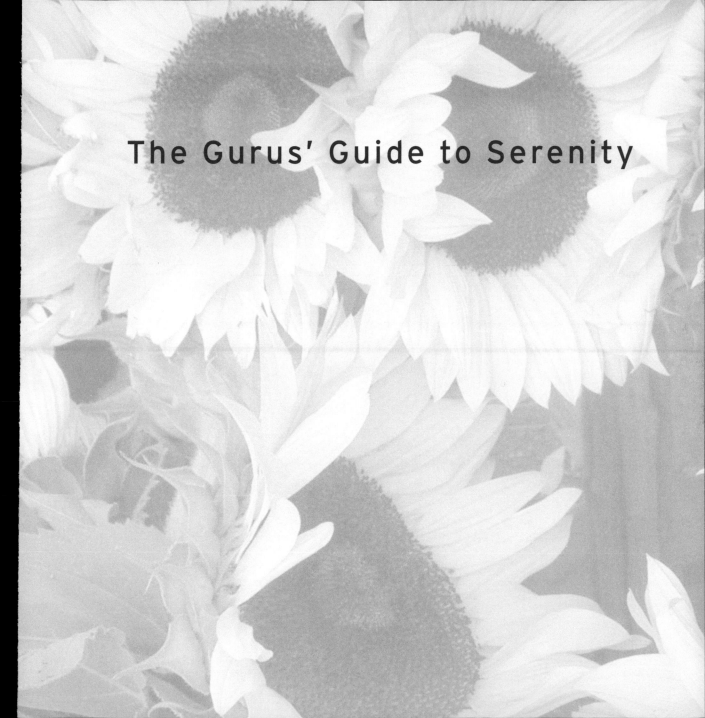

The Gurus' Guide to Serenity

Chapter One

Savor Your "Me-Time"

WE ARE LIVING in a time of fast-paced over-achieving. Rushing through our days forces us to rush through our lives, and all too frequently we miss the most important, yet simplest details that make us truly happy. Baths, spa treatments, massage, yoga, meditation, cooking, art projects, gardening, knitting, sacred spaces, stretching, relaxing, and breathing deeply are often completely overlooked and undervalued.

We have been raised with the mantra that we can have and

accomplish anything and everything, if we work hard enough. This concept, though common today, may still be a bit foreign to our mothers or grandmothers, many of who were raised to raise and born to breed. They were praised for their Bundt cakes, perfect children, and sparkling floors. They were ladies who lunched and kept themselves well groomed. They adored their husbands and cherished their children. In fact, they very well may have doted on their kids a little too much, maybe even to the point of imposing, because as the 1960s progressed, many young, blossoming women set themselves "free."

Being a housewife was suddenly "out," and free loving was "in." But when the realization took over that the hallucinogenic heydays were coming to an end, many women traded their tie-dyed shirts for suits. They quickly dismissed the role of the 1950s housewife and explored every crevice of political and economic freedoms that had for so long been denied to them. The feminist movement was birthed, and soon these women, briefcases in hand, invaded the predominantly male working world. For many, housekeepers were hired to facilitate the abandoned role of the mother, creating a new variable in the family unit—the nonkindred caretaker.

Women today want to have it all. We, the "do everything" women of the twenty-first century, want to raise our own children while continuing to make a substantial financial contribution to the family, pleasing our spouses, maintaining friendships, and simultaneously being happy ourselves. Impossible? Maybe. But we certainly persist. For most of us, this equation of life can be a little daunting, with the ultimate result being an overextended, overwhelmed, ostensibly flaky woman. We end up spending so much time trying to do and be everything that we forget to be ourselves. We overlook the most important, though seemingly insignificant details, like nurturing our spirit and our soul. So where does this leave us? In a constant state of crisis.

Midlife crisis is no longer solely a term used to describe men in their fifties who suddenly realize that everything they have accomplished has not produced the happiness and fulfillment they had expected. Unfortunately, "do-everything" women are also experiencing midlife crises. Instead of running off and buying expensive cars, getting tattoos, or leaving their spouses for their secretaries, women are feeling emptiness and a longing for times past. Having spent a lifetime nurturing our children and pleasing our bosses, employees, and co-workers, we are in dire need of nurturing and bettering ourselves. Giving ourselves permission to take a "time-out" is an issue for many of us who have always catered to the needs of others. In our moment of crisis, we are realizing that we have spent our lives living to work and not enough time working to live.

But it is not just those of us in our fifties who are in a crisis situation. New terms have been created to describe the confusion, depression, and instability of children who have been caught in the crossfire. Those girls, turned women, are our friends, daughters, or maybe ourselves. We have graduated from college with the mantra ingrained in our heads that we can be anything and do everything. And many of us are shocked by the reality of life. We have new fears and doubts about relationships as our parents or friends' parents get divorced, a harsh reason that our own "happily ever after" often fails along the way. Some young women expect to find successful careers that pay enough money to purchase a house and a car immediately. We are all too often way too keen to be all grown up, which manifests in jump-started marriages that quickly crumble, careers that prove unsatisfying, and a sense of self that seems to be diminishing. We have fallen into the "quarter-life crisis."

While self-help books are fine, at the age of fifty or even twenty-five, we are tired of being preached to and promised to be "saved." We need more than to hear that stress is bad and finding time for ourselves is good. We need, instead, real-life tips, advice, and suggestions on *what* we ourselves can do and *how* we can do it to achieve a stressless, or at least less stressed life.

Celebrities are often the barometers for what is "hot." And though their lives are filled with glitz and glamour, even celebrities need a break, a moment's rest that is purely for themselves. It is personal time minus the Hollywood boyfriend, the manager, the agent, the makeup artist, the paparazzi, and even the fans. Celebrities work so hard to maintain their perfectly sculpted outward appearance, but sometimes, like us, they need a little inner nourishment as well. From yoga to knitting and the dependable bubble bath, celebrities somehow find ways to work alone time into their jam-packed schedules. Although some celebrities are able to conjure up calm on their own, most need a little guidance from their "gurus." From personal trainers to aestheticians, yoga experts to aromatherapists and herbalists, these purveyors of serenity offer celebrities spiritual and emotional health and well-being while helping them develop the creative outlets that nurture the soul.

The Gurus' Guide to Serenity is a compilation of some of the tips and advice that gurus give and celebrities receive. So as you begin to read this book, take a deep breath, relax, and enjoy some "me-time."

Chapter Two

Beauty and the Bath

Preparing for a bath is like setting
the table for a five-course meal.
— TAG GALYEAN

Blissful Baths: The Powerful Potion of Water

Baths have been a mode of pleasure, relaxation, and ritual since the Romans and Greeks discovered the delights of both hot and cold bathing. Every culture has its own bathing preferences and practices. In some societies, taking a bath is merely an infrequently used method of cleansing the body. Other traditions use the power of the bath's waters to rebirth or purify the body of sins. Some swear that baths are therapeutic and vital to health, while others have taken the practice of bathing to an art form. But regardless of religion, custom, or status, it is clear that baths are both physically and emotionally cleansing.

I must admit that bathtime is my (Laurel) favorite time. It is my time to be alone in a candlelit room, soaking in warm, bubbly water as my body sinks into a tensionless state of bliss. I have a drawer filled with bath crystals, oils, bubbles, and potions that are added to my tub according to my mood and needs of the moment. But no matter what my mood may be, I find that I always crave a bath. Whenever something stresses me out, or I am lonely or sad, my first thought is, I need a bath. Instinctually, I want to wash away my troubles and feel comforted and immersed in a tub of warm, healing water. I also take baths before bed to ensure a restful night's sleep, soothe sore muscles, and simply relax amid fluffy bubbles and sensual scents.

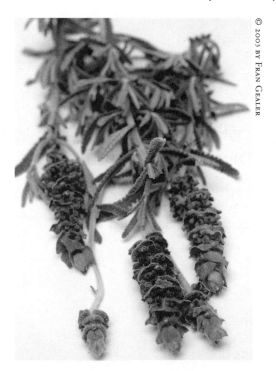

© 2003 BY FRAN GEALER

Think about it: Baths take us back to a time when we had little or no stress, when we didn't even know that stress existed! Water makes up 75 percent of our bodies, 90 percent of our blood, and 85 percent of our brains. Our first nine months of existence were spent in a womb of warm liquid. We used to play in the bath with our toys, making bubble beards and mustaches on our faces to amuse Mom and Dad. Those were the good old days. We looked forward to bathtime back then because it was fun. We look forward to bathtime now because it is relaxing. Baths are inexpensive, easy, convenient, and totally destressing, yet often overlooked and undervalued.

Allow your body to relax and feel completely at ease and soothed as you submerge yourself in a bathtub filled with warm, comforting water.

Tag Galyean's Perfectly Designed Bath

Baths have the potential to be playgrounds for the senses. Tag Galyean, an internationally recognized spa and pool designer, creates these luxurious playgrounds at spa resorts worldwide. His TAG Signature Spa provides guests with a physically and emotionally therapeutic experience. Tag creates an utterly healing and restorative spa oasis by bringing together a perfect balance of technologically advanced therapies and time-tested remedies. Turnberry Isle, Hotel Hershey, La Quinta, the Broadmoor, and the Greenbrier, all resorts known for their spas, are just a few of his clients. Baths are one of Tag's specialties; as he explains, "Cocooned in warm water, in a darkened space, all body parts gently surrounded and held absent of stress and fear, you are able to experience the ultimate self-kindness, centered around the element of 'me'—my body, mind, and soul." Baths are naturally calming as they relax the nervous system, calm the muscular structure, and allow quiet time with the self. There is an innate sentiment of safety when submerged in bathwater, which allows you to let down your guard and release stored stresses.

Tag equates a bath to a dinner: "Preparing for a bath is like setting the table for a five-course meal." There are many considerations to take into account, including water temperature, lighting, music, and additives like bubbles, salts, and oils.

The temperature of the water plays an important role in a bath's relax-

Tag's Recipe for a Revitalizing Morning Wake-Up Bath

Set the water to a cool temperature.

Add a few drops of
Rosemary
Pine

Soak and wake up!

ing effect, explains Tag. "There will be an exchange through the skin of bath minerals flowing into the body and toxins moving out from the body. Temperature balance is important to this flow. Start with water at 100 degrees Fahrenheit (water that is too hot will drain and exhaust you, while it will overstimulate if it is too cool)." In order to make certain that what is flowing into your body through your skin is pure, use purified water whenever possible. Now that the temperature is set to satisfaction, it is time to create the mood.

More than a tub filled with warm water, there is often a soothing ambience that helps in the creation of this relaxing ritual. Sights, sounds, and scents all play into the overall appeal of a comforting bath. Some of you may choose to paint your walls calming colors, others adorn countertops with scented candles and photos of your loved ones, and still others ease the mind and body through music. "The physical environment is of great importance to the bath experience," explains Tag. "Light, color, sound, air

Tag's Recipe for a Restful Nighttime Bath

Set the water to a warm temperature.

Add a few drops of
Lavender
Ylang-ylang

Soak and slow down.

quality, and air temperature are all playing a part." Paint the walls of your bathroom a color that is soothing to you. For some, that may be a creamy yellow, while others prefer a lovely lavender or sky blue. Candles, incense, or freshly cut flowers will infuse your bathroom with sensuous smells. Mozart or Marley playing in the background can mimic or help modify your mood. And so, the atmosphere is complete!

You can enhance the water's benefits by filling your tub with a variety of skin-nourishing, protecting, detoxifying, energizing, relaxing, or moisturizing ingredients. The offerings are wide-ranging and include anything from age-old kitchen remedies such as milk, cream, oatmeal, or salt to today's more sophisticated bath supplements, such as essential oils, sea algae and seaweed, caffeine, or concentrated seawater pumped from the ocean's depths, which provide an assortment of benefits, including softening skin, relaxing muscles, calming the mind, reducing cellulite, boosting energy, pacifying inflammation, and remineralizing the body. You can

Tag's Recipe for a Refocusing Bath After a Stressful Situation

First, wash in the shower.
Soak in hot water.
Add sea minerals.

even take advantage of the natural resources from your region. If you live in California's Napa Valley, known by many as "wine country," fill your tub with grapes and reap the antioxidant rewards. A native to Hershey, Pennsylvania? Try a chocolate facial that is both tasty and skin quenching. Is your hometown deep in the heart of Wisconsin? Soak in a milk bath. If the desert state of New Mexico is where you reside, take a trip to your backyard and snip a stem of aloe vera. The juice is a natural skin healer and moisturizer. Live in the Garden State of New Jersey and had a bumper crop of cucumbers this year? Be creative. Thinly slice an extra one and place it over your closed eyes for a quick pick-me-up.

Sometimes the bathtub itself can play a role in the stress-relieving success of bathing. Are you soaking in a claw-foot tub or a spa tub filled with jets? Tag's specially designed baths take place in flow-through or overflow soaking tubs. As in infinity pools, the bathwater in these tubs is constantly flowing over the sides in a steady stream. A cast-iron claw-foot tub may take you back to bygone times, when life was easy and traffic jams were nonexistent. While you may want to luxuriate in the old-world style, many of the claw-foots of today are equipped with back-massaging, bubble-making jets. You can choose from simple tubs or deluxe tubs that can easily fit four. There are tubs with seats on the side in case you want to take a momentary breather, heart-shaped tubs, even tubs with home-theater, surround-sound entertainment systems (complete with floating remote controls). Bathing has been thrust into a new level of indulgence!

Celebrities often have the fortunes to indulge in life's most luxurious "me-time" delights, yet countless celebrities treasure their bathtime above all else. Baths have the power to melt away stress and bring you back to yourself.

Susan Lucci's "Bring Me Back" Baths

Susan Lucci's daily bubble baths are her "me-time." This actress on *All My Children* lives an incredibly time-crunched life. Her days are strewn with demanding schedules and filled with travel, early call times to the set,

Susan's Recipe for a "Bring Me Back" Bath

1 bathtub filled with warm water
Invitation Bath Gel bubbles
The soothing sounds of Latin or jazz music

Steep for 15 to 20 minutes, 5 nights a week.

press tours, meet-and-greets, interviews, autograph signings, and special appearances that can leave her feeling rushed and harried (though you would never know it from her grace and constantly friendly demeanor).

At the end of the day, the last thing she wants is to follow any sort of an agenda. Her nightly bathtime ritual allows Susan time to return to herself and relax. She fills her tub with her own bubble bath creation, called Invitation Bath Gel, which is packaged and sold for at-home use. "Baths bring me back to me. They make me feel like a girl again," she says. As Susan basks in her bubble bath, she listens to the cool sounds of Latin or jazz music. She explains, "I play Latin or jazz music and relax in a luxurious tub filled with bubbles for fifteen to twenty minutes. It is amazing how those few minutes can do so much."

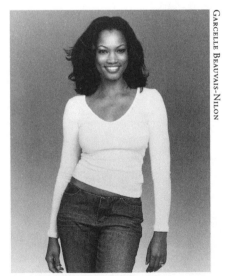

Garcelle Beauvais-Nilon

Garcelle Beauvais-Nilon's Bathroom Sanctuary

For the *NYPD Blue* star Garcelle Beauvais-Nilon, destressing is a "work in progress." It is about taking time out to be completely in the moment. Whether she is simply walking down the street and appreciating the surrounding flowers and trees or reveling in sumptuous spa treatments, Garcelle has learned to indulge in "me-time." Like many other celebrities, she seeks serenity in the healing waters of a bath. In fact, her bathroom is designed to be a warm haven, a private sanctuary in which she delights in girlie pleasures like makeup and scented baths.

Baths are known for their sedative effects. In fact, it is believed that steeping in a warm bath for ten minutes before bedtime will promote a more restful sleep. Garcelle takes full advantage of the relaxation-inducing warmth of the bath just before bed.

Lisa Rinna's Bathtub Built for Four

The *Days of Our Lives, Melrose Place,* and *SoapTalk* star Lisa Rinna has created a sacred space for herself within her bathroom, a room that her actor husband, Harry Hamlin, built. After a hard day of work, she is sometimes able to steal a few minutes for herself in her bathtub built for four, to calm her nerves and ease her mind. Lisa says, "I have a little 'me-time' every day,

Lisa's Recipe for a Blissful Bathroom

1 bathtub built for four

Candles. Lisa loves Slatkin & Co.'s large floral-scented candles.

Mineral bath salts. Whole Foods Market has one of Lisa's favorites: Batherapy in Green, which costs only $7.

Family photographs in beautiful frames

Cozy robe

Classical music

10 to 20 minutes alone

even if it's eleven at night, I always have privacy in my bath. I love baths because they feel great and they relax me after a hard day of work or parenting. They literally wash the stress away." Though the tub is wonderful, especially in the early evening when the sun peeks in through the windows, it is the collection of family photographs in beautiful frames arranged alongside that adds a personal touch. Lisa fills the bath with scented suds and the room with the soothing sounds of classical music to create an environment of complete calm. Within ten or twenty minutes, her two daughters can't stand even one more second of mommyless time, so they often bounce into the tub with her.

Teatime in the Tub

Tame your tension, soothe your soul, and mend your mind with tea in the tub. Drinking tea can be incredibly calming and relaxing. Imagine the utter indulgence of bathing in it! The healing properties of tea have been depended on for health and wellness for thousands of years. Steep your body in a bath of rose petals. Melt away your tension with stems of lavender, or indulge in the intermingling of lemongrass, orange peel, and ginger. You can buy premade tub-size tea bags called Tub Tea or create your own tea bags using cheesecloth, or any porous cloth or material, and a string. Fill the cloth with your desired herbal concoction, tie the ends together, and soak away your stresses in a giant tub of tea.

Morning Rise and Shine Tub Tea

Fill the tub with 85°F water. Setting the temperature on the cool side will keep you from falling back to sleep while stimulating, reviving, and cleansing.

Add dried herbs or essential oils of peppermint, juniper, and/or eucalyptus. You can either fill a homemade bath tea bag with dried herbs or drop 5 to 10 droplets of the essential oil in the tub as the water is running. Peppermint cools and rejuvenates the body and spirit with its tingly sensation (for a colorful morning bath use crushed, fresh peppermint leaves). Juniper is energizing and stimulating as well as a natural astringent. Eucalyptus is stimulating, protective, and a disinfectant and decongestant whose powerful scent prevents tired eyelids from closing.

Take 15 to 20 minutes of soak time to cleanse and rejuvenate.

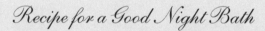

Recipe for a Good Night Bath

Fill the tub with 95° to 100°F water. The warm water will soothe the mind and muscles, preparing the body for a good night's sleep.

Combine dried or fresh rose petals or their oil, a pinch of crushed cloves, and lavender essential oil in a homemade bath tea bag. Rose, celebrated for its promotion of love and compassion, will help combat insomnia and release tension. It is extremely gentle and calming, even for the most sensitive skin. Clove has been used in various traditions for its soothing and healing effects. Lavender, an incredibly mild essential oil, calms and reduces tension.

Bath pillows are great cushions for the head and neck.

Dim the light or use candlelight.

Soak for 20 to 35 minutes to rest and relax.

Soothing Foot Soaks

The average person walks approximately 100,000 miles in a lifetime, which translates to four times around the earth! That is a lot of pounding on the precious seven thousand nerve endings, twenty-six bones, 107 ligaments, and nineteen muscles that make up the foot. So why don't we care for our feet with even a quarter of the money and time we put into maintaining our cars? It is time to nurture the feet that so diligently and reliably transport us.

A long, hard day of work, running around in high heels and rarely allowing yourself a moment to sit, can wreak havoc on your feet. A bubble bath, or simply a basin filled with warm water and healing herbs and oils, is all you really need for foot pampering. If you are not a bath person per se, or you're just not in the mood tonight, a footbath is the perfect quick

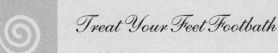

Treat Your Feet Footbath

1 big bowl
Warm water to fill ¾ bowl
Dried sage or essential oil of sage
Dried rosemary or essential oil of rosemary
1 teaspoon almond oil
2 tablespoons nonfat dry milk
5 to 15 minutes of soak time

fix. Simply steep your feet in healing waters for approximately fifteen minutes and, voilà, refreshed and happy feet! There are tons of fabulous premade footbath formulas, such as Get Fresh and Bath & Body Works, but you can just as easily make your own. So relax and relieve your swollen feet as they soak in steamy water filled with healing remedies. Your feet will tingle with happiness.

RESOURCES

www.tagstudio.com
www.wholefoodsmarket.com
www.getfresh.net
www.bathandbodyworks.com

Chapter Three

Your At-Home Spa

All you need is the mindfulness
that you are a sanctuary unto yourself.
—*Jillian Wright*

Facials, Body Scrubs, and Other Beauty Treatments

When someone says "spa," what images come to your mind? Total relaxation, blissful pampering, white terry-cloth robes, soapy, scented water, flickering candles, and gobs of moisturizer are just a few of the thoughts that dance in my head and attract me and millions of other women to spas. Spas represent the ultimate indulgence. Unfortunately, not only are they indulgent in terms of making us feel like pampered princesses but they can also levy quite a tax on our time and our pocketbooks. It's easy to drop hundreds of dollars and several hours on a treatment. Well, guess what, you can create a spalike atmosphere in your own home for pennies!

If you have five minutes or five hours, with a few added spalike details, you can evoke the smells, sights, and sounds of your favorite sumptuous spa. Ready to relax? Dim the lights and fill your house, or at least your "spa room," with the warm flicker of candles. Buy a few bunches of sweetly scented flowers, such as roses, gardenias, Casablanca lilies, tuberoses, or lavender, and allow the aroma to soothe your mind. Turn on a CD of jazz or the sounds of nature, and relax. Create your own refreshing spa drink by adding a few cucumber slivers, lemon slices, or orange wedges to a chilled glass of water. Don't forget to turn off your phone. The stinging ring can immediately transform the soothing spa you have worked so hard to create back into a regular old room. Spend a day at the spa, called your home . . . indulgences included!

Glow—Where the "Upper Crust" Go

Glow Skin Spa in New York City is where the upper crust relax and revitalize, and are utterly pampered. Fortunately, we too can enjoy the indulgences of Glow Skin Spa, thanks to its owner Jillian Wright's favorite at-home spa recipes!

Jillian believes that "you don't need a fancy spa to destress your life." While her spa is a pleasure chest for celebrities like Alicia Silverstone, Ivana Trump, Téa Leoni, Lisa Loeb, and Gabriel Byrne, all of whom are in desperate need of a little coddling, Jillian encourages many of her clients to pamper themselves in the comfort of their homes with homemade treatments similar to those professionally administered at the spa. Little preparation is needed, and a whole lot of pleasure is accomplished. All you need is hot water, some creams and potions, fruits and vegetables, and a few deep breaths, and you are on your way to your at-home spa.

You can create your spa in your bedroom, garden, bathroom, or any sacred space that allows a few minutes of peace and quiet. Jillian teaches her clients that "all you need is the mindfulness that you are a sanctuary unto yourself. Just be sure to acquire quality 'me-time' to make your life more meaningful and valuable." One day you may choose to pamper yourself with a facial. Another afternoon, you may want to give a little extra loving to your fingers and toes. Or you may simply choose to sit in a candlelit room and sip on some spa water. Regardless of your spa treatment selection of the day, enjoy your time away from the real world and simply relax. You can even luxuriate in your at-home spa with a lover or friend and trade off giving treatments to each other.

Sometimes we take for granted the healing and restorative power of simple touch. Remember way back when, when you refused to fall asleep at night unless your mom gently rubbed your back? What about those five minutes when the hair washer at your favorite salon massages your scalp as she works in the shampoo and conditioner? It is as though the gentle fingers touching your head or body have the power to turn off the stresses and frustrations of the day. Restorative touch is an important aspect of Jillian's job and something that she believes is an essential element to a healthy life. "There is nothing like touch. Touching in a nonsexual way is rare and much needed to sustain balance in your life. This can be in the form of a massage, a pedicure, cuddling, or hugging. Touch ultimately has the power to heal a wounded spirit."

So turn off the television and prepare to be pampered!

Though most of you probably already have sitting in your refrigerator, pantry, or medicine cabinet the majority of ingredients for the following at-home spa treatments, here is a shopping list you can use:

Exfoliating mask	Tomato
Chamomile tea	Parsley
Moisturizer	Lemon
Mud mask	Egg white
Mango	Oatmeal
Avocado pit	Rosewater
Orange zest	Lavender essential oil
Organic cocoa	Rose petals
Honey	Rose essential oil
Cream	Mint oil
Oat flour	Chamomile flowers
Cottage cheese	Fresh peppermint
Avocado	Eucalyptus oil
Potato	Cucumber
Eye cream	Orange
Horseradish root	Lime
Plain yogurt	

We all look forward to vacation time! With spa treatments you can elicit a vacation state of mind without getting on an airplane. Oftentimes spa treatments have the ability to transport you to another place and time. As you doze off into a world of total relaxation and bliss, your thoughts

Glow Skin Spa's Recipe for a Stress Reduction Facial

Create a relaxing ambience—light candles and listen to soothing music.

Apply an exfoliating mask (most of you will have some sort of exfoliating mask in your box of beauty tricks).

Over a pot of hot water infused with chamomile tea or eucalyptus oil, steam your face for 5 minutes (the mask should still be on).

Remove the mask with a warm washcloth.

Gently, in a circular motion, massage a rich moisturizer onto your face.

Gradually apply more pressure in areas of stress (wrinkles will often reveal stressful sections), such as your forehead, between your eyebrows, and your temples. This mini massage will help improve circulation and open your sinuses.

Apply a clay or mud mask to release impurities.

Relax for 15 minutes as the mask dries.

Clean your face with a cool washcloth.

While taking deep, cleansing breaths, apply a light lotion to your face.

Smile.

begin to float away and the lines that distinguish fantasy from reality blur into a pleasant haze. The scent of the mango or warm coconut oil that is being massaged into your shoulders, or the subtle sting of the sea salt that you scrub into your skin allows your mind to wander back to some romantic island retreat you had years ago. Distant images reemerge as you envision yourself in that relaxing moment, on the beach, beside your loved one. Spa treatments are more than a good rubdown, exfoliation, or pustule excretion. They are like mini-vacations that can heal the body, mind, and spirit.

Spa treatments can be more indulgent than you think. In fact, several include delicious ingredients like chocolate, whipped cream, and honey. Talk about decadence! Many foods that you find in your refrigerator or pantry are filled with skin-soothing, cleansing, exfoliating, and moisturizing properties.

Chocolate, when rubbed on your skin, is incredibly indulgent yet completely guilt-free. It is also aromatherapeutic. Think about it: Many of us

Glow Skin Spa's Recipe for a Virgin Gorda Mango Body Polish

1 ripe mango
1 tablespoon crushed avocado pit
1 tablespoon orange zest

This is a great body polish because it is easy and fun to do! Avocado is excellent for dry skin and is also rich in antioxidants. Just save your avocado pit from the guacamole you made the night before! Wash it off, put it in a ziplock bag, and crush it into pea-size pieces. Let it dry overnight on a cookie sheet. The next day, grind the avocado pit in a coffee grinder or food processor and mix it with the mango and orange zest. Voilà! Spread the mixture all over your body in the shower. This will get the blood circulating and the antioxidants running rampant.

Glow Skin Spa's Recipe for a Chocolate Fondue Facial Mask

½ cup of organic cocoa
¼ cup honey
4 tablespoons heavy cream
3 teaspoons oat flour
3 teaspoons cottage cheese
3 teaspoons avocado

Mix all the ingredients together and apply to the face, neck, and chest. In addition to the benefits mentioned in the text, oat flour contains beta glucan, which has antiaging properties. This mask promotes blood circulation, so expect it to feel tingly after about 5 minutes. Leave it on for 15 minutes, then rinse off (perhaps in the shower with your loved one)!

first experienced aromatherapy when our moms were baking chocolate chip cookies. Suddenly we were overcome by a sense of ease and happiness. Chocolate naturally provides a feeling of elation. More than mental therapy, it has an incredibly high concentration of antioxidants (comparable to black tea and red wine), as well as tons of vitamins A and E. When all is said and done, chocolate is good for your skin and good for your soul. So why not rub it all over your body? Cream, cottage cheese, whipped cream, and milk are extremely effective exfoliants because of their lactic acid. They soften, soothe, moisturize, and tighten the skin.

Glow Skin Spa's Recipe for a Raw Potato Eye Mask

Looking a little worn down? Are your eyes strained from too many hours staring at the computer screen? Apply a little tater, and your eyes will brighten up in no time!

Peel and grate a raw potato.
Mix it with your favorite eye or facial cream to make a mask.
Apply to delicate eye areas and leave on for 15 minutes.

The potassium in the raw potato will temporarily lighten nonhereditary dark circles.

Stimulating Horseradish Hair and Scalp Treatment

¼ cup finely grated horseradish root (you can also use horseradish from the jar)
¼ cup of plain yogurt

Mix the two ingredients to form a paste, and massage it into your hair.
Wrap your hair in plastic for 15 to 20 minutes, then shampoo and rinse.
The horseradish stimulates blood flow to the scalp, which helps prevent hair loss.

Tex-Mex Arriba Arriba Facial Mask

½ small tomato
¼ cup fresh parsley
1 teaspoon lemon
1 egg white (optional)

Make sure you use fresh ingredients. Do not use store-bought salsa, because its spices and peppers may irritate the skin.

Combine the tomato, parsley, and lemon in a blender until pureed.

Add the egg white afterward, if desired.

Apply to your face for 10 minutes. Rinse off with warm water. Follow with your favorite moisturizer! You can refrigerate the rest of the mask if you want to use it later in the week.

This is an excellent recipe for oily, stressed-out skin!

Honey is an antiseptic with natural cleansing properties as well as a humectant, drawing moisture to the surface of the skin. Suddenly, you will find that you view your kitchen in a whole new way!

Most of us already have chocolate, milk, and honey conveniently stored in our refrigerators and pantries. So pull them out and follow the recipes below and your skin will reap the rewards. It will save you a trip to the spa!

If you are surprised by the fact that chocolate is food for the skin, what would you think if I told you that potatoes, horseradish, tomatoes, and parsley are also unbelievably skin satiating? Well, they are! Potatoes are filled with potassium, which lightens and brightens the skin. They are particularly great for dark circles around the eye area. Horseradish stimulates the scalp and is therefore excellent for those of us with thinning and receding hairlines. Tomatoes seem constantly to be in the media as their health benefits continue to be unveiled. Now we recognize that they are good for the face too! Tomatoes contain great quantities of lycopene, which is known for its antiaging and antioxidant properties. When they are blended with parsley and lemon, the result is a slightly acidic combination that is perfect for decongesting and balancing the skin. Lemon is also a skin lightener and can help balance areas of hyperpigmentation.

Amber Valletta's Beauty Secrets

Amber Valletta is paid to be beautiful. Her supermodel status allows her to travel the world posing for the camera. While seemingly glamorous, constant travel can truly take a toll on the body and mind, leaving the skin and attitude dry and irritated. Yet Amber appears to be unaffected by her jet-setting lifestyle because she fills her spare moments with various forms of "me-time." Spa treatments are certainly a favorite. "I love massage. I love facials. I even like getting waxed. I just love any sort of spa treatment!" she says. Oftentimes the mere thought of a spa can provoke a calming effect. Because Amber is exposed to such an array of spa opportunities in the cities and countries she travels to, she tries to take advantage of treatments indigenous to the area that she has never before experienced.

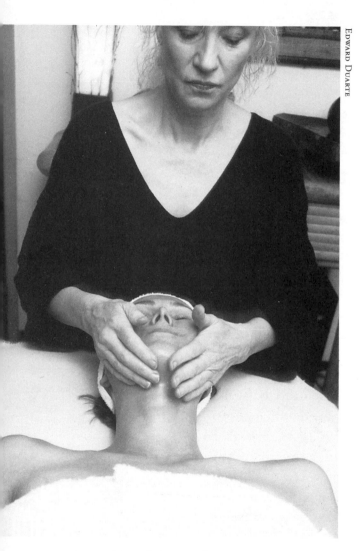

EDWARD DUARTE

Arcona giving a face-contouring massage.

Arcona* Unveils Inner Radiance

Touted by many as "the facialist to the stars," including Madonna, Lauren Graham, and Diane Lane, Arcona, who owns a skin-care line and a luxurious spa in Los Angeles, is a firm believer in the absolute necessity of treating yourself to daily "me-time" indulgences. But these indulgences should not be viewed as excesses; "me-time" is essential to your health and well-being. Arcona deems anything that destresses the body and improves the function of the internal organs "me-time." Decreasing stress and lifting the spirits make the body and mind healthier. Spa treatments do more than relax your mind and body; they also help to beautify and unveil inner radiance and a natural glow.

Celebrities, in particular, should indulge in "me-time" spa treatments because, explains Arcona, "their faces are their fortune." Lauren Graham enjoys both Arcona's spa offerings and her at-home skin-care products. She declares, "I

*Arcona recently passed away. However, the Arcona Spa, under the direction of Chanel, continues its tradition of natural beauty.

love all of Arcona's products, as well as the facial-contouring massage, which will leave your face glowing!"

Many of Arcona's treatments are rooted in Chinese medicinal practices and the belief that your face reflects the inside of your body. Arcona's facials help break down and flush out the stress the face retains. "We carry a lot of stress in the face," she says. "For the body, we exercise to reduce stress. My treatments exercise the face and therefore relax the body. It is like yoga. Every time you exercise a facial muscle, it relieves tension."

We constantly use our facial muscles. When we smile, laugh, talk, frown, or raise an eyebrow, we are flexing our facial muscles. It is interesting that more muscles are used to smile and laugh than to frown. This is because it is more difficult to lift the cheeks and corners of the mouth against gravity than it is simply to allow the face to droop. Your mother used to tell you that if you made an ugly expression, your face would freeze that way. Well, in a way, she was right! Over time, the lines, creases, and wrinkles that are left will come to reflect years of smiles, frowns, and

Arcona's Facial Exercises

Sit on the floor with your knees bent, your behind resting on your calves.
 Stick out your tongue as far as possible.
 With your tongue still out, open your eyes as wide as they will go.
 Hold this funny face for several seconds.
 Completely relax your eyes, mouth, and jaw.
 Repeat at least 5 times.

Arcona's Multiple Uses for Yogurt

Yogurt is amazing for your skin. It is filled with lactic acids and milk proteins that moisturize and firm the skin.

For a yogurt facial or body facial:

Apply a generous amount of plain yogurt to your face and body. Use
    approximately 2 cups for your body and ½ cup for your face.
Let it sit for 20 minutes.
Rinse.

For a yogurt bath (remember that Cleopatra used to take milk baths):

Mix about 3 cups of plain yogurt into a warm bath.
Let your skin lap up the nutrients for 30 minutes.
Repeat once a week.

furrows of the brow. In other words, your personality will be permanently ingrained on your face. So start smiling!

Arcona helps to ease stubborn lines before they become permanent reflections of you. She explains, "It is said that by age forty your face reflects exactly who you are through the laugh lines, worry lines, sad lines, and anger lines. Though I think that the lines between the eyebrows are not worry lines, they are thinking lines. People who don't have lines between their brows make me wonder if they have done much thinking throughout their lives!"

Aside from being aware of the emotions your face echoes, Arcona says it

Arcona's Recipe for One of the Easiest Masks on Earth—The Honey Mask

In the "olden days," people used honey to heal wounds. Honey is filled with healthy bacteria and enzymes that dissolve dead cells and other debris from the skin. It is like a hydrogen peroxide and a natural humectant that draws moisture to the surface of the skin. Honey is extremely rejuvenating and will simply make your skin glow.

Apply a generous portion of honey to your face.
Massage into the skin for several minutes.
Rinse.

is possible to care for your skin in a way that makes you appear ageless: "When you take care of yourself in a natural way, using natural products, your skin remains radiant and glowing. That is what beauty is. And every magnificent moment you spend pampering and caring for yourself can and should be considered your 'me-time.'"

Garcelle Beauvais-Nilon's Favorite Facial

On a television soundstage, the lights can be blinding. So when Garcelle Beauvais-Nilon is off the *NYPD Blue* set and ready to relax at home, the first thing she does is dim the lights. Light has the power to set a mood. It can make us uncomfortably alert, as when we are sitting in a dentist's chair. Or it can put us peacefully at ease, as when we are watching the moonlight reflect off the ocean. When giving yourself an at-home facial (if you aren't planning on torturing your skin with extractions), turn down the lights and allow your mind to unwind.

Garcelle loves facials. And when she can't get to a spa, she does them herself with her facial in a jar—Bioelements clay mask. Though it frightens her son, she loves to walk around the house as the mask hardens on her face. And when she removes it, her skin is refreshed, revitalized, and ready to face the harsh lights on the set the next day!

Even Fitness Experts Find Time for Their Faces

Kathy Kaehler, the fitness expert for the *Today* show and celebrity trainer, with high-profile clients such as Julia Roberts and Claire Forlani, is also a mother of three who leads a bicoastal life. She is always in search of a little time for herself, and the way she keeps it all together is weekly "me-time" facials and foot massages. Sheryl Lowe, Rob Lowe's wife, referred Kathy to the facialist Nerida Joy, and now Kathy can't live without her. While having her face rubbed and relaxed by a professional is always an indulgent treat, with kids, work, and countless prior obligations, it's often difficult for Kathy to find the time to escape for a few hours. So she has come up with her own at-home facial that is just as relaxing, doesn't require an appointment, and is much more convenient.

Kathy Kaehler's Recipe for the Perfect Relaxing Facial

Plan a play date for the kids at someone else's house!

Add a drop of essential oil to 3 cups boiling water. The type of oil depends on your mood and what you need (lavender to relax, rose to soothe, or peppermint to uplift).

Steam your face for 5 to 10 minutes.

Rinse with warm water.

With your fingers, gently apply a mixture of egg whites, ground oatmeal, and rosewater. (The consistency should be like a heavy liquid.)

Sit or lie down and relax for 15 minutes.

Gently remove the mask.

A Soothing Steam

Steaming is an incredibly simple yet utterly indulgent spa treatment that de-stresses, detoxifies, and moisturizes. If your preferred travel destination is a humid rain forest, you will love this at-home treat. Either fill your bathroom with the steam from your shower or just fill a pot of hot water and place your face a few inches above it. Allow the moist heat to open your pores, eliminate oils and impurities, cleanse, soothe, and moisturize your skin. Add a few herbs like lavender or rosemary and further increase the benefits. Or go out to your garden and pick a few roses for your steam treatment.

Many of us are naturally drawn to roses. Of course, we love to get them as gifts from suitors, display them on our dining room tables, grow them in our gardens, and even wear their scent on our skin. Yes, the rose certainly has found its place in women's hearts. But more than merely a fragrant flower, the rose is a symbol of love, sensuality, and compassion. Its healing scent helps to release anger and stress, minimize PMS and insomnia, fight infection, heal eczema, and promote cell rejuvenation. No wonder we are naturally drawn to roses!

Lavender is another one of those miracle plants that we have loved for centuries. Even the Royals have been known to "need" lavender. Charles VI of France was said to require lavender-filled pillows. Queen Elizabeth I of England apparently demanded lavender preserves and fresh lavender sprigs at Her Majesty's table. Evidently, Louis XIV bathed in lavender-scented water. And Queen Victoria supposedly kept her scent sweet by smearing herself with lavender deodorant. Lavender is also said to treat restlessness, insomnia, fungus, flatulence, bacteria, and airborne mold; it has even been shown to be useful against impotence. In fact, a study revealed that pumpkin and lavender were the aromas found most arousing by men. With this lengthy list of benefits, I'd say it's time to place a lavender-filled pot in every room in your house!

With the use of a few natural products, you can transform a simple steam into a decongestant, eye-opener, or sleep inducer in just a few minutes.

Tracee Ross's Favorite Beauty Secret

As the daughter of the world-renowned singer Diana Ross, the actress Tracee Ross entered naturally into entertainment. While her acting career on *Girlfriends* is certainly important, Tracee has decided to incorporate vacation time into her daily life rather than wear herself so thin that a two-week vacation becomes essential (the way most of us vacation). She takes daily vacations through her various modes of "me-time." She emphasizes "various" because she says that she "gets really bored really fast." But, her favorite destressing indulgence is steaming. She says, "Steaming makes me feel so refreshed. I have a steam shower bath in my house, and I use it so

A Soothing Steam

Steamy hot bath or bowl filled with water
5 drops of lavender essential oil
Handful of fresh rose petals or buds
3 drops of rose essential oil

Allow the ingredients to steep for 5 minutes.

Steam for 5 to 10 minutes while seated in the bathroom or with your face over the bowl and a towel over your head to collect the steam.

Pat your face with a cool washcloth to close your pores and refresh your skin, bringing you back to your senses.

Liberally apply moisturizer.

A Decongestant Facial Steam

Steamy hot bath or bowl filled with water
5 drops of mint oil
Handful of dried chamomile flowers
Handful of dried peppermint leaves
3 drops eucalyptus oil

Allow the ingredients to steep for 5 minutes.

Steam for 5 to 10 minutes while seated in the bathroom or with your face over the bowl and a towel over your head to collect the steam.

Pat your face with a cool washcloth to close your pores and refresh your skin, bringing you back to your senses.

Liberally apply moisturizer.

often that sometimes I wonder if it is possible to steam too much!" She puts honey all over her body, then steams the toxins and impurities out of her skin. Yes, it can get a bit sticky, but, as we've seen, honey will leave your skin looking silky smooth and revitalized.

Healing Spa Water

Water . . . drinking it can be just as renewing as bathing in it, as long as it has the proper fixin's. What is the first thing you are offered upon entering

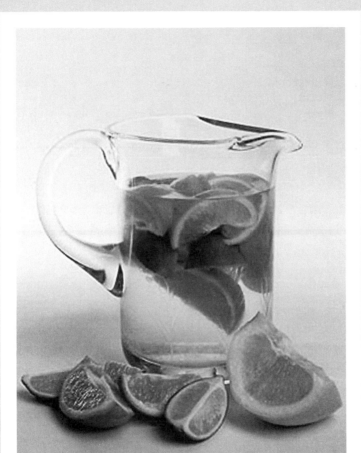

Simple Spa Water

1 jug of cold water
Generous amount of ice
Sliced cucumbers
Sliced oranges
Sliced lemons
Sliced limes

Combine.
Stir.
Ahhhhhhhhh!

a spa? Ice-cold water with hints of fruits, vegetables, and herbs is customary within the spa culture. Naturally flavored waters are an essential component to create a spalike feel. From cucumbers to mint, oranges, lemons, and limes, spa waters evoke an immediate sense of calm as your body and mind prepare to relax or come back to reality before and after a pampering session or just because you feel like having a refreshing drink.

Susan Lucci's Quenching Healthy Habit

The *All My Children* star Susan Lucci appreciates the hydrating and revitalizing benefits of water, especially spa water. She practices the healthy habit of "drinking at least eight glasses of water throughout the day," even more if exercising strenuously and regularly. She says, "Since drinking water can be boring, sometimes I spice it up with a spritz of lemon or lime or cucumber for a refreshing alternative. Water is also very important for muscle tone, both in the body and in the face." You wanna really glow from the inside out? *Hydrate!*

• • •

With a few simple ingredients, which you probably already have tucked away in your refrigerator, pantry, or even growing in the garden, your house can instantaneously transform into your personal relaxing sanctuary! Cucumber water, herbal facials, and sumptuous steams are perfect individually or combined and can provide a relaxing spalike experience. If only that handsome spa therapist were part of the deal! Oh well. . . . That's why we are equipped with very active imaginations!

RESOURCES

    www.unwind.com is the place to unwind online
    www.glowskinspa.com
    www.arcona.com
    www.bioelements.com

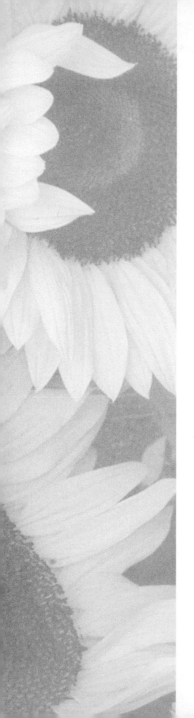

Chapter Four

Massage . . . The Need to Knead

If there is a puddle of drool on the floor
when the massage is done, I know it
was a success.
—LAUREN HOLLY

MASSAGE HAS LONG been recognized for its healing and soothing effects. In fact, in 100 B.C., Julius Caesar was known to be "pinched" every day, as he used massage therapy to relieve his neuralgia and epileptic seizures. Beyond the positive physical and emotional responses conjured by massage, it is simply pleasurable. In fact, there are few things in life that I (Laurel) enjoy more than an oil-slathered, full-body, deep-tissue massage. Not much compares to a good ol' rubdown.

Good Ol' Rubdown

Massage should be included as a monthly "me-time" ritual. More than a luxurious way to unwind, massage has several health benefits. In addition to relaxing the muscles and promoting a sense of calm, massage has been proven in various studies to improve mood, quality of sleep, immune system function, and sex drive, and to reduce anxiety, fatigue, headaches, and upset stomachs. So make an appointment at your nearest day spa and indulge! If you are uncomfortable walking around nude among other lounging ladies, the indulgent alternative is to bring the massage therapist to your home! Celebrities treat themselves to the luxury of an in-home massage on a regular basis for privacy and sheer convenience.

Lauren Holly's "Me-Time" Luxury

Many celebrities select several types of "me-time," depending on their mood, location, and shooting schedule. The actress Lauren Holly, known for her roles in *Dumb & Dumber, Any Given Sunday,* and *What Women Want,* is certainly no stranger to the need to destress after a long day of film cameras, bright lights, and paparazzi. But Lauren is convinced that "you can never get away from everything. It all started with call waiting. Now, no matter how hard you try, you are always accessible through cell phones, pagers, and so many other things." She used to feel selfish about taking time out for herself, but now Lauren realizes that "me-time" is essen-

RACHEL BATI

Lauren Holly

tial. She says, "I am convinced that I look younger, feel healthier, and I know I'll live longer now that I allow myself time to relax."

One of Lauren's favorite "me-time" luxuries is massage, particularly if it's from someone who she knows and feels comfortable with. "Massage is a given," she says. "Once you get one good one, you want more and more." Oftentimes massage therapists will begin the treatment with some talking. They may ask questions about what your body needs, where you are sore, and what type of pressure you prefer. Sometimes the chitchat carries into the massage a bit. But Lauren's favorite part is when the talking stops and she is allowed to doze off. As she says, "If there is a puddle of drool on the floor when the massage is done, I know it was a success."

Michelle Kluck's Magic Fingers

The massage therapist Michelle Kluck has spent the past ten years kneading the stressed muscles and sore feet of celebrities such as Salma Hayek, Joe Pesci, Ashley Judd, and Sigourney Weaver. "Everyone's feet are the mirror of their body," says Michelle, and massage provides a great way to escape the worries of the day and take a mini break from everything. Even a five-minute chair, neck, or foot massage is beneficial. Michelle views massage as a truly perfect "me-time" activity, because "it is a time when you can, and should, tune everything and everyone out and focus on yourself. It's the time when you can turn inward and pay attention to your own needs. During a massage, you can give yourself a break from the 'chatter' in your head and just let go. It's your time to space out and relax your body and your mind." Massage induces physical and emotional healing of the body, mind, and soul. A few of the benefits include the following:

Massage Benefits for the Body

- Relaxes the body and calms the nervous system
- Lowers blood pressure and reduces heart rate
- Increases blood and lymph circulation
- Stimulates the removal of waste and toxins in the body
- Loosens tight, aching muscles and stretches connective tissues
- Strengthens the immune system
- Lessens chronic pain
- Reduces tension headaches and the symptoms of PMS
- Stimulates the release of endorphins, the body's natural painkillers
- Relieves cramps and muscle spasms
- Increases flexibility and range of motion
- Promotes deeper, more effective breathing
- Speeds recovery from illness
- Improves skin and muscle tone
- Reduces swelling and scarring
- Increases tissue metabolism
- Improves posture and decreases muscle deterioration

Massage Benefits for the Mind

- Reduces mental stress
- Promotes better sleep
- Encourages mental relaxation
- Improves concentration

Massage Benefits for the Soul

- Reduces anxiety
- Encourages healthy body awareness and positive self-image
- Enhances creative expression

Celebrities love to relax under Michelle's healing hands because, she explains, "in addition to the many stress-relieving physical and psychological benefits, massage can enhance creative expression." As we know, acting is an extremely creatively demanding career. "Oftentimes, when you calm your body and quiet your mind," says Michelle, "you allow yourself to open up to new ideas and thoughts. After a relaxing massage, many celebrities have told me that they can focus better, everything becomes clearer to them, and they can feel a creative flow."

Think about it. Are you one of those people who comes up with brilliant ideas in the shower or just before you fall asleep at night? I sure am. The reason is that you are momentarily not thinking about work or all the crazy things happening in your life at that second. You are finally allowing yourself to let go and relax. And when you are relaxed, your mind is able to think more clearly, allowing creative thoughts and ideas to emerge seemingly "out of the blue." It is the same with massage. While deep in the moment of my massage, I find that I remember all the things I have forgotten to do. I come up with inspired ideas and perfect solutions . . . but then I get so relaxed I pass out. When the massage is over, I am fully aware that I had a ton of extraordinary revelations, I just can't remember what they were! Maybe next time I will bring a pad of paper and a pen with my robe and slippers!

Michelle's clients request her presence around the clock and around the country. She explains, "Celebrity clients often have crazy schedules, and their only free time for 'me-time' might be late at night or very early in the morning. I try to accommodate them as much as possible, whether it's on set, in their trailer, or in their hotel room. During filming, celebrities may have fifteen-minute breaks, so you have to be ready for when they get a few free moments to relax. I also try to leave them with something that they can use to destress themselves when I'm not around, such as peppermint lotion that they can rub on their temples and neck or an eye pillow to help them fall asleep."

The Healing Foot Rub

Though it would be nice, few of us can afford a regular full-body massage by a professional masseuse. But don't worry, your hands can be taught the correct kneading techniques and pressure points to bring bliss to yourself. Back massages are wonderful but hard to do on yourself, so it's a good thing that feet are great recipients for massage as well! More than just conveniently placed and easy-to-reach, feet are known as the "gateways to the body." And considering the fact that we walk an average of seven miles per day, you can always use a foot massage. Foot massage, or reflexology, is actually an ancient practice of manipulation and stimulation to restore health and balance to the entire body. In holistic healing tradition, it is believed that the foot is the mirror of the entire body. Through massaging the feet, it is possible to bring the body into bal-

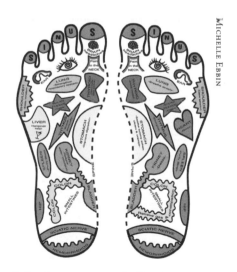

Reflexology massage socks diagram.

ance. Rapidly growing in popularity as an alternative and complementary method of healing, reflexology allows you to rub your own aches, pains, and stresses away. The actress Lauren Holly loves her foot rubs. "If you don't have the time for a massage, then get a foot massage. I love them!"

Michelle's healing hands can't get to everyone, so she developed massage cure-alls for when you don't have a masseuse at your disposal—Reflexology Sox and Reflexology Shirts, which allow those in need of some kneading to massage their own pains away. The Sox are great because they show you exactly where to knead your feet to relieve anything from headaches, an upset stomach, or PMS to insomnia, anger, or even sexual dysfunction. It is amazing what your own two hands can do!

Michelle's Basics for an At-Home Massage Regimen for the Feet

Keep your hands soft. In order to strengthen your body's own healing abilities and soothe your body and mind through reflexology, you need to maintain a soft, healing touch.

Be aware of sensations. If you find a sensitive area, reduce the pressure. Reflexology massage is supposed to feel good.

Feel it. Really try to feel the foot. Don't just rub according to protocol and technique. Instead, use your fingertips to detect subtle changes. You may find that some areas feel grainy and others are soft and supple. The "grains" are crystalline calcium and uric acid deposits that can block the free flow of energy throughout the body. Spend a few moments gently massaging these areas. But be aware that they may be more sensitive.

Allow your intuition to kick in. While maintaining the intention of healing, allow your fingers to move around the foot as they please. They may be drawn to areas of congestion, which signal potential problems in the corresponding organ. A congested area may manifest as warmer or colder than other spots.

If your feet are ticklish, try to apply steady, direct pressure to reflex points. Usually, the ticklish feeling comes from light, feathery touches. A firmer touch will minimize the tickle response.

Michelle's Foot Reflexology Techniques

Creating warmth: Rub your hands together to build some warmth.

Holding: Cradle one foot in your hand for a few seconds as you take a couple of deep breaths.

Supporting hand: Use one hand as the "supporting hand" and the other (usually your dominant hand) as the "working hand." This helps you to stabilize the foot and apply the appropriate amount of pressure.

Rotation: To warm the foot fully, hold the heel with your supporting hand and use your working hand to rotate the ankle in each direction. Next, take each toe and roll it in either direction. This increases blood flow in the feet and begins to relieve neck and shoulder tension.

Stretching the Achilles tendon: Cup the heel in your supporting hand and flex the toes back and forth with the working hand. Then flex the entire foot back and forth and allow it to awaken.

Loosening the ankle: Place both hands on the soles of one foot so that your pinkies touch down the middle of the foot. Gently rotate your hands, moving the ankle side to side. Loosening the ankle joints loosens all the joints in the body.

Kneading: Using both thumbs, knead the sole to improve circulation. Work your thumbs from toes to heel and back.

Thumb crossing: Hold the foot with both hands. Place your fingers on the top and your thumbs on the sole, resting your thumbs horizontally against each other. Applying steady pressure, slide your thumbs across each other, side to side, working your way up and down the sole.

V thumb slide: Place your hands in a similar position as in the thumb crossing. Beginning at the heel and in the middle of the foot, with alternating thumbs, press out and up the foot in V formations.

Static pressure: By applying steady, static pressure to specific reflex areas, you can relax particular body parts. Inhale while applying pressure. Exhale and release. You can also rotate your finger on the reflex point for a more pulsating pressure.

Thumb walking: Hold the heel with your supporting hand and place your working thumb on the desired reflex point. Slowly move your thumb up the foot in an "inchworm" movement. Always walk the thumb forward, never backward.

Finish: When you have completed your foot massage, using your fingertips, imagine that you are brushing off negative energy, lightly moving from the heel to toes. Then, brush the top of the foot from the ankle to the toes. Wrap both hands around the foot and hold for several seconds.

Michelle's Five-Minute Anxiety-Releasing Foot Rub

Sit down and take off your shoes.

Knead the brain, stomach, and solar plexus points on the feet.

The brain is crucial to ease the mind. Knead the point at the base of the ball of the big toe to target the brain.

Rubbing the stomach area on the foot, located at the arch, helps relieve anxiety-related "butterflies."

The solar plexus is the "nerve switchboard of the body." The coordinating spot is in the center of the base of the ball of the foot. Work your finger magic by pressing into the solar plexus spot for 20 to 30 seconds on each foot. Repeat. Grainy or tender areas may represent imbalances of energy. By concentrating the massage in those areas, you can release the blockage and restore a healthy balance.

Drink a glass of water after your foot rub to flush out released toxins.

Michelle's Foot Rub to Reduce Insomnia

Sit down and take off your shoes.

Knead the brain, thyroid, pineal, pituitary, and solar plexus points on the feet.

Stimulating the brain helps ease your mind of the day's stresses. Knead the point at the base of the ball of the big toe to target the brain.

The thyroid works to stabilize hormones. Rub the crease that connects your big toe to the ball of your foot and you have found your thyroid.

Massaging the pineal gland point regulates your sleep cycle while promoting a more restful slumber. Beside the brain, along the top of the inner edge of the big toe, is the reflexology equivalent to the pineal gland.

Working the pituitary gland encourages relaxation and balances energy levels. The pituitary gland point is just below the pineal gland point. Walk your fingers to the base of the inner edge of the big toe and you will have stumbled upon the pituitary gland.

Rubbing the solar plexus point relaxes the nerves and calms the whole body. The solar plexus point is in the center of the base of the ball of the foot.

Drink a glass of water after your foot rub to flush out released toxins.

Fall asleep.

Stress Reduction Brow Massage

Many of us scrunch our brows when we are stressed. Repetitive scrunching causes wrinkles and piercing headaches. For a quick fix that you can do anytime, almost anywhere (except maybe in a business meeting), using the pads of your index fingers, pinch your eyebrows firmly for several minutes and feel the tension slip away. There are great products that you can use in addition to your fingers' pressure to help alleviate the tension, such as Origins' Peace of Mind On-the-spot relief.

Stressful Jaw Breakers

After a long night's rest, you would expect to rise revitalized. Unfortunately, for many of us, this is not the case. We often wake up with headaches, and the funny thing is that our jaws feel just as exhausted and sore as our heads. Yet another unfortunate by-product of stress is grinding your teeth and clenching your jaw during sleep. Doesn't stress ever take a break? To find out if your jaw may be the root of those frustrating morning headaches, clench it and feel the muscles that surface on either side. Are they oddly sore? You may not even have known that those protruding muscles existed. Gently massage the tender area with your fingertips, and it just might relieve your headache. Since we have a hard time controlling our jaw movements while asleep, you can purchase a mouth guard from your pharmacist, or ask your dentist to mold one specifically for your mouth. It may cost you a couple hundred bucks, but to avoid that type of debilitating headache, it is worth it (and your liver will thank you too, for cutting down on your pain reliever consumption).

• • •

Another alternative to an expensive spa day or at-home massage is a visit to a massage chair. These wonderfully relaxing and soothing chairs are finding their way to health expos, health food stores, and yoga centers. Sometimes for as little as a dollar a minute, a technician will give you a mini massage, working the shoulders, back, arms, and neck. Many Whole Foods Markets stores now feature the chairs at their entrances.

RESOURCES

Hands on Feet by Michelle Kluck
www.basicknead.com
www.origins.com
www.wholefoodsmarket.com

Chapter Five

Finding Your Bliss Through Yoga

*The power of yoga [is its ability] to open
people up, allowing them to let go and
quiet down.*
—BRYAN KEST

YOGA, THE SANSKRIT WORD for union, is the creator of calm for countless celebrities, including Cindy Crawford, Amy Smart, Gwyneth Paltrow, Christy Turlington, Jolie Fisher, and, of course, Madonna. Within the seamless movements of yoga, there is a spiritual element that helps to center, balance, and unite the body and mind. Through fluid yet precise and controlled exercises, each part of the body is relieved of built-up tension. While it is a method of relaxation, yoga is also recognized as one of the best ways to transform the body into a slim and toned vision of perfection, while simultaneously exercising the mind. In fact, several celebrities have given up traditional forms of exercise altogether, swearing that yoga is all they need to keep their bodies svelte and healthy.

This ancient art is now imparted through countless instructors, books, and videos. Blossoming from its roots millennia ago, yoga has transformed into a proliferation of styles, each of which has its own speed, pace, and approach. A few of the disciplines include Anusara, Ashtanga, Bikram, Hatha, Integral, Iyengar, Kundalini, Power Yoga, Tantra, and Vinyasa. Undoubtedly, one of these styles will suit your needs and desires.

Anusara is a heart-focused discipline that uses biochemical principles in an attempt to achieve the optimal blueprint for each individual body through a combination of flowing movements and long holds. *Ashtanga,* meaning "eight limbs," emphasizes the continuous and synchronized flow of the breath and bodily movement using six scripted sequences of postures with twenty-five to forty postures in each. *Bikram* classes follow a precise series of twenty-six movements practiced in rooms that reach 105° Fahrenheit in order to obtain a deeper stretch and mental concentration while sweating out impurities. *Hatha* literally means "moon (*ha*) and sun (*tha*)." *Hatha* refers to the basic and elemental principles of yoga and the physical movements, postures, and breath work that help to maintain physical, mental, and spiritual balance. Anusara, Ashtanga, Iyengar, and Power Yoga are actually rooted in Hatha yoga. *Integral* is a more breath-based style that also incorporates chanting and meditation, achieving a deep state of relaxation. *Iyengar* consists of a precise and alignment-focused series of poses that are held until they are "fully experienced." *Kundalini,* a metaphor to describe the flow of energy and consciousness within us, is a quick, stimulating, strengthening, and centering yoga practice that consists of breath work, poses, chanting meditation, and fast, repetitive movements. *Power Yoga* is an intense and flowing style that encourages you to work hard sensitively while concentrating on proper breathing and moving through a series of postures that make your muscles work and body sweat. *Tantra,* contrary to common Western belief, is not merely a sexual practice. Instead, it helps to stimulate awareness and break down mental barriers and self-imposed blocks through poses, chants, and breath work. *Vinyasa,* arguably the most popular yoga practice in the United States, links breath work with a series of flowing movements.

While each practice is called "yoga," the various twists on this age-old tradition allows students to select the technique that best fits their personal style. Whether your ultimate motivation for practicing yoga is spiritual, physical, or a combination of both, there is a yoga practice to suit your needs. Within each style, you will experience a unique "me-time" sensation. It is easy to find yourself transported and transformed during your yoga experience, unable to concentrate on anything but the moment. You are keenly aware of every detail of your body's inner and outer movements. While practicing yoga for one hour a day may be optimal, just ten minutes can effectively rejuvenate your mind and exercise your body.

Total Fitness for Your Body and Mind at Kundalini Yoga East

Marisa Tomei, Ian McKellen, and Helen Mirren unwind and relax through meditation and yoga at Kundalini Yoga East, a haven for stressed-out New Yorkers. Amid bustling New York City, Kundalini Yoga East is a respite of tranquillity, allowing students to unwind and spend a period of time focused solely on themselves. Classes create an invigorating and inspiring setting. Students emerge refreshed and revitalized and can achieve total body and mind fitness, healing emotional and physical stresses including headaches, anxiety, depression, and sleeplessness, while burning calories, toning the body, and balancing their metabolism.

Kundalini Yoga East's Recipe for Yogic Aspirin: Left Nostril Breathing

Relieve headaches without popping pills with Yogic Aspirin.

Sit in a relaxed position.
Press your right index finger against your right nostril, plugging the airway.
Breathe deeply and slowly through the left nostril for 3 minutes.
You will feel a cool, soothing breath flowing in and out of the nostril.

Kundalini Yoga East's Recipe for Yogic Valium: Meditation on the White Swan

Experience the destressing benefits of Valium the way the yogis have for hundreds of years.

Sit with your spine straight in a comfortable, cross-legged position.

Make fists with both hands.

Raise your fists with the backs of the hands toward you, 6 to 8 inches directly in front of your brow point.

Extend and press your thumb tips together until they become white (do not press hard, just firmly).

Let the last joints closest to the tip of your thumbs relax and bend, the tips facing down.

Fix your eyes on your white thumb tips.

Close your eyes and mentally see your thumb tips.

Begin to take long, deep, slow breaths.

On the inhale say to yourself, *"Sat,"* and on the exhale say to yourself, *"Nam."* *Sat* means "truth," and *Nam* means "identity." Combined, *Sat nam* means "Truth is my identity."

Repeat for 5 to 11 minutes.

Kundalini Yoga East's Recipe for Yogic Ginseng

Get an immediate and lasting burst of energy.

Sit with your spine straight in a comfortable cross-legged position.

Roll your tongue into a V with the tip just outside your lips.

Inhale deeply through your rolled tongue.

Exhale through your nose.

Repeat for 2 to 3 minutes.

Kundalini Yoga East's Recipe for Yogic Fountain of Youth

Maintain a youthful exuberance.

Sit with your spine straight in a comfortable, cross-legged position.
Place your arms at your sides, elbows pointing down, with your forearms per-
pendicular to the floor and upper arms parallel to the floor.
Have your palms face each other at the level of your head with fingers pointing up.
Alternate moving your arms up and out at a 60-degree angle and then back to the
original position as though you were slicing through the air above your head.
Do this as fast as possible, breathing with the movement.
Work up to 6 minutes.

Kelly Rutherford's Girl Time

When you get stressed and tired, sometimes it is difficult to pinpoint the root of your stress. The actress Kelly Rutherford, known for her role as Megan Lewis Mancini McBride on *Melrose Place,* star of "Threat Matrix," as well as countless other TV and movie roles, has come to the realization that she needs regular girl time in order to destress. Actually, it is her boyfriend who came up with that conclusion. When she is in a bad mood, he often asks, "When was the last time you had any girl time?" Girl time, for Kelly, is her "me-time," be it a yoga class, getting her nails done, or being involved with a women's group. She says, "You almost have to make sure that you take the time to schedule it. Your girl time doesn't always have to be the same activity; it depends on what you are in need of at that moment."

Kelly, along with several other celebrities, is involved with Step-Up Women's Network, a nonprofit organization that is committed to empowering women and girls to make positive social change in our society through philanthropic and networking functions as well as professional development programs, community outreach, and mentorship opportunities. The group is particularly known for activities such as Step-Up for Yoga and Health, one of Kelly's favorites. Tons of women, from all walks of life and with a multitude of interests, descend upon the recurring yoga event and stretch their minds and bodies for a good cause.

Alicia Leigh Willis Cleanses and Energizes

Alicia Leigh Willis makes sure that she stays serene on the high-strung *General Hospital* set by regularly stretching her body and mind in yoga. She explains, "We put our bodies through so much stress, and yoga is a great way to heal. After you are done, you feel cleansed and energetic." Alicia practices Ashtanga yoga, which allows her to go beyond her limitations and experience a new radiance. As she says, "I do things with my body that I never knew I could do. The handstands are great to do in the morning because the blood rushes to your head and it really wakes you up! Sometimes, I have to get up at 4:30 to start shooting *General Hospital,* and a handstand gets me going that early in the morning." Handstands are definitely positions for more advanced yogis. For less advanced yogis, Alicia suggests, "You can stand on your hands against the wall. Hold it for thirty seconds or so. Then, gently release your legs back down to the floor." Once you gain more confidence and control, you can work your way up to a full handstand without a wall for support. Soon you will find no need for that first cup of coffee, because a handstand can be safer and more effective than a caffeine buzz.

Power Yoga to Quiet the Mind

Establishing "me-time" is the essence of Power Yoga—creating an "empowering experience through yoga." It is also an intense workout for the body and mind. Bryan Kest, the founder of Power Yoga, feels that the duty of a yoga instructor is to create the right environment for "quieting the mind." He believes in "the power of yoga to open people up, allowing them to let go and quiet down." Though based in Los Angeles, Bryan travels the world to introduce novices to the power of Power Yoga. His goal is to get students out of their heads, giving their brains a little rest from the incessant input and output that normally is passing through. Clearing the stress from minds and bodies allows for an essential moment of rest. Even the American Medical Association acknowledges that 80 percent of disease is stress related, a huge figure that can be greatly reduced.

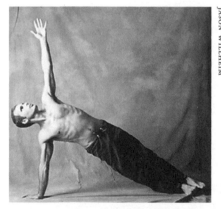

JASON WILLHEIM

Bryan Kest of poweryoga.com in a Power Yoga pose.

If you ever have a chance to get to one of Bryan's Los Angeles Power Yoga classes, you will find yourself dripping in sweat shoulder to shoulder with some of Hollywood's

Bryan Kest's Recipe for the Beginner Power Yogi

First, you must make the commitment in your own mind . . . a commitment to yourself. We sometimes have to get to a point where we are so stressed out that we force ourselves to make room for something like this.

Make yoga a part of your schedule.

If you can't find a class or are still a bit intimidated, try a videotape. There are many to choose from.

biggest celebrities. Many people fail to realize that celebrities experience bad days, breakups, breakdowns, weight problems, and stress, and deal with the same fears and insecurities that we all do. Yoga helps celebrities get out of the "all about me" state and into balance.

While Bryan is considered a guru by many, he realizes that the information he is spreading is not new. In fact, it is ancient. Still, he feels blessed that he has been given the opportunity to help people. The tools that he teaches motivate others to get started in their own yoga programs of self-healing.

USA Today reported that an estimated fifteen million Americans practice yoga. While yoga is unbelievably popular, many people still have not experienced its power. It is easy to declare, "I really need to start taking a few yoga classes." But oftentimes we will repeat that statement for years, fearing the initial class. To fear the unknown is natural; I did it (Laurel). My mom (Sharon) gave me a ten-class yoga pass as a Christmas gift. I held on to it in my wallet (just in case I suddenly felt the urge to go) for an entire year before finally getting up the nerve to take the first class. Of course, I was immediately hooked, and before I knew it, those ten classes were long gone and I had purchased an unlimited pass.

Mahshid Tarazi's Sumo to Stretching

Mahshid Tarazi is the North American female sumo wrestling champion in the Women's Heavyweight Division. She also placed fourth in the world, the only American to place among thirty-eight competing countries, and she will participate in the Olympic Games. Mahshid is also a Power Yoga devotee. She says that Power Yoga helps her on many levels, both in life and in her sumo wrestling career: "Sumo is all about balance. I fight women who are three hundred to four hundred pounds, more than twice my size. In order to be competitive, I must maintain my balance and concentration. That is my biggest strength. I maintain my stance. The audience calls me 'the girl with the heart' because I'm the smallest competitor in my category and I stand my ground. I have a lot of heart. I want it, and I push to the end." The concentration she practices in yoga helps Mahshid live for now. She explains, "When you are competing, [living in the moment] is such an essential component for success. It is also about perseverance. When it is tough, you push through to the end. Yoga is very complementary, as it teaches you to push through sometimes awkward or uncomfortable positions, offering serenity on the other side. Yoga also helps me release pressure. I use it when I'm doing sumo, but also in my everyday life. Releasing pressure through meditation gives me endurance.

When I am fighting people who are bigger than I am, they get tired faster than I do.

Mahshid takes Bryan's class three times per week as part of her training routine. Her mom also uses Bryan's tapes, though she never actually goes to class. "In class," says Mahshid, "I am focused and I feel reborn, and cleansed. I can handle life better. Every time that I go to class, [it is very difficult, and] I wonder if I can complete it. Once I get started, I wonder, How could I not have? While yoga can be a mental break and an emotional time-out, the practice does not always come naturally. You have to train your body and mind in order to hold the difficult poses and not give up when you feel uncomfortable. Many yoga poses require a great deal of strength and balance. Both are achieved and increased, but only with perseverance."

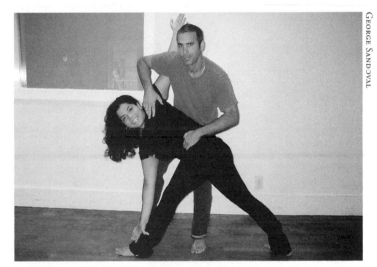

Bryan Kest and student Mahshid Tarazi.

Janet Gunn Rids the Chatter

The *Silk Stalkings* star Janet Gunn says, Power Yoga "takes away the chatter from my head—the voices telling me you can't do that. When you are running through your day [in your head], listing all the things that you have to do, all of those things keep you from living in the moment, yoga takes away that chatter and allows you to live in the present." Practicing Power Yoga two to three times per week is teaching Janet how to live in balance, dedicating time to her family, her jewelry company, and her acting career.

Anna Getty's Yogic Awakening

One might think that growing up a Getty, Anna Getty was virtually born with a silver spoon in her mouth, one that, like many elite offspring, she carried into her adult life. Yes, for a while, she frequented the hottest Hollywood galas and get-togethers, socialized with other elite offspring, and caused a ruckus all over town. In her words, she was "an insane mess, filled with fear." But Anna had always been a seeker and a traveler, a trait passed down from her mom, and she quickly discovered yoga. Anna's yoga practice began much like many others; in fact, much like my own. She drove by the famed Golden Bridge Kundalini Yoga Center in Los Angeles, owned by the celebrity yoga guru Gurmukh Kaur Khalsa, picked up a schedule, and promised herself that one day she would make it in there. Well, days turned to weeks, weeks to months, and she still hadn't mustered the courage to enter this unknown territory of Zen-like Angelenos toting yoga mats. Finally, she took a class, and the flood of emotions that were released manifested themselves as tears. Anna knew her life was about to

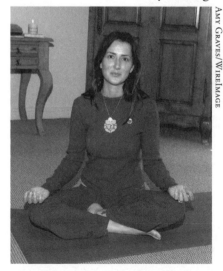

AMY GRAVES/WIREIMAGE

Anna Getty practicing Kundalini Yoga.

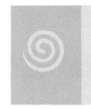

Anna's Favorite Healing Mantra

"Happy am I, Healthy am I, Whole am I"

change. For a while, she tried to uphold her party girl lifestyle, showing up to class after only a few hours of sleep and still brandishing glitter around her eyes from the night before. The nightly partying and drinking had left her body in a state of toxic shock, but the yoga was helping rid the toxins and change her behavior patterns as her body was awakening and regenerating. She felt as though it was time to make a choice: continue on this new path or go back to the Hollywood scene. She chose the yoga.

Soon, Anna was traveling with Gurmukh. Her life was changing before her eyes. She found that she was becoming more forgiving, patient, and flexible in both her body and her life. The next step was to take the teacher training class in order to share her new love of yoga by teaching others. Now she and her husband have a meditation room in their home, a room for spiritual and emotional growth, for healing and expression, or for simply sitting still.

RESOURCES

www.kundaliniyogaeast.com
www.stepupwomensnetwork.org
www.poweryoga.com
www.goldenbridgeyoga.com

Chapter Six

Meditation—Relax and Say "Om"

*Learning to observe experience from
a place of stillness enables you to relate
to life with less fear and clinging.*
—ANN BUCK

THE ANCIENT PRACTICE of meditation has its roots in many Eastern religions and was popularized in America during the 1960s by Maharishi Mahesh Yogi. Still revered and explored for its healing and calming effects, meditation, once primarily a religious practice, has been adapted to fit our fast-paced lifestyles. Meditation is a mental exercise that helps us shelve old habits, remove the mind from a frazzled and overwhelmed condition, and create inner peace and a healing state of calm. Meditation is not a religion; it is a healing technique. Just like golfers practice their swing at driving ranges to improve their games, people who meditate get mentally, spiritually, and physically in shape to live life more healthfully. Meditation allows you to remove your inner critic and focus on the here and now, without letting your mind wander in destructive directions.

More and more, meditation is being incorporated into conventional medical approaches, fortifying the benefits of modern medicine. Some doctors even prescribe meditation. This individualized practice uses natural resources that best suit a person's body, basic skills, mind, and schedule. While there is substantial documented proof that meditation effectively yields a myriad of physical and emotional benefits, the fact remains that if you tell the average athlete that he or she needs to meditate and/or do yoga in order to speed up recuperation from an injury, he or she may do it for a few days, but then will most likely lose interest and stop. As with any skill, meditation takes time to learn and adjust to. It takes patience, trial and error, and maybe even a few lessons to get the basics down and begin to enjoy meditation's rewards.

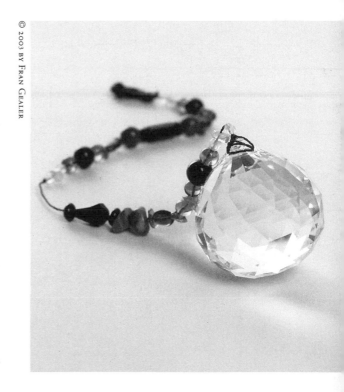

While most people think of meditation as simply sitting in a dark room with eyes closed and legs crossed, there are actually many types to choose from. Meditation can take the form of a morning walk through the neighborhood, during which you allow your mind to be free from the daily stresses of

Five-Minute (or Less) Meditations

CALMING MEDITATION

Close your eyes. Slow your breath. Concentrate on the sound of the inhale through your nose and the exhale through your mouth. Breathe deeply, using your diaphragm. Breathe in for a count of 3, lightly hold for a count of 3, and exhale slowly and steadily until you have emptied your body of air for a count of 3. Repeat at least 5 times. Now allow your breath to go back to its natural rhythm.

MIND'S EYE

Focus your eyes on a peaceful object for a minute or so. Now close your eyes but continue to envision that object in your mind's eye. As you breathe in, maintaining the image in your mind, think happy thoughts. Next, exhale all negative thoughts. You can also do this exercise visualizing colors. With closed eyes, imagine that you are breathing in pure white (new and positive thoughts) and breathing out black (stale and unhappy thoughts).

EXERCISE

Physical activity allows your mind to be as free and uninhibited as your body. Experiencing raw and unbridled energy through exercise can elicit a euphoric meditative state, such as "runners' high."

life. It can also be participating in your evening yoga class, spending time in your garden, or taking five minutes to step outside your office building during a hectic day. You can meditate almost anywhere, as long as you allow your mind to be free from negative, stress-inducing thoughts. Practicing the type of meditation that is natural to your body and captures your skills and interests will increase the chances that you will follow through and dedicate yourself.

The basic goal of meditation is the creation of a feeling of interconnectedness, a sensation of serenity that allows us to traverse the storms of stress. Even if you don't feel change at first, keep putting in the effort, and eventually you will carve away at the stalwart rock that we call stress.

Basic Meditation Techniques

Each form of meditation uses concentration techniques to help us stop our minds from wandering. Once the mind is calm, we have the ability to achieve a state of serenity and balance.

Concentrative Meditation

Transcendental Meditation (TM) and Kundalini are two types of concentrative meditation during which you focus on a mantra—a word or phrase that is chanted out loud or internally. Transcendental Meditation has origins in ancient Vedic tradition preserved for many generations by a long line of teachers in the Himalayas. The TM technique is secular, subscribing to no particular religion, belief, or lifestyle. You can easily learn TM

from an experienced instructor. This form of meditation is almost effort-
less, requiring only the act of sitting quietly, eyes closed, in a comfortable
chair for twenty minutes each morning and night to relax and refresh. The
daily routine of TM generates more noticeable effects as tension and stress
are released, increasing vigor and intellect. The unique state of restful
awareness imparted through the practice of TM allows the body to reach
deep tranquillity while the mind dissolves accumulated stress and utilizes
dormant creative potential. This state can stimulate your motivation, vi-
vacity, and latent energy, which may enhance your contentment and success in your daily life.

Insight or Mindfulness Meditation

Also known as Vipassana meditation in the Buddhist tradition, insight
meditation has been practiced in Asia for more than twenty-five hundred
years. This simple meditative practice focuses and calms the mind by allowing its subject to become acutely aware of his or her thoughts and sensations in order to overcome negative and unhealthy habits. Much of
insight meditation consists of silent observation. As Ann Buck explains,
"Learning to observe experience from a place of stillness enables you to relate to life with less fear and clinging." Through observation, you can gain
the ability to see life as a constantly changing process and accept its ups
and downs without getting caught up in them. Insight meditation is a tool
to train, stabilize, and purify the mind. To try insight meditation, sit cross-
legged, completely still, eyes closed, in silence, with your mind's eye focused on your abdomen. Be aware of the movements of your belly. Your
mind will travel to a more concentrated state.

Expressive Meditation

Expressive meditation shatters the assumption that meditation requires sitting in silence. Rather, this form of meditation involves movements designed to release physical, mental, and emotional stresses. It is a non-threatening and completely familiar form that includes dancing, twirling, shaking, jumping, laughing, humming, and simply making random noises combined with movement. This free-flowing technique helps to unleash creative energy and spontaneous passion. Though they often seem silly, these actions can, in fact, ignite deep healing and enhanced self-awareness. Allow yourself to get "caught up" in the moment and soon your mind and energy will uncoil, releasing self-imposed blocks that may have hindered emotional growth. This is the perfect meditative practice for the hesitant new meditator.

Ways to Get Started with Expressive Meditation

JUGGLING

Juggling requires unwavering concentration to keep the balls in the air as opposed to on the floor. Start with two balls. Then try three. With practice, you will get into a rhythm, a state of flow, during which your mind is so integrated into the activity that you stop dropping the balls. Eventually, you can achieve a degree of mindfulness during which you have awareness of sensory information (sight, sound, smell, touch, and perception) while simultaneously being cognizant of your thoughts and emotions. This is a state similar to what many athletes refer to as "the zone."

PAT AND RUB

Another fun, mind-activating endeavor is the seemingly simple task of simultaneously standing on one foot, patting the top of your head with one hand, and rubbing your stomach with the other hand. It takes coordination, concentration, and a comfortable floor (in case you fall over). Ultimately, you can reach a total mind-body connection and meditative state with this simple exercise.

VISUALIZATION

Imagine yourself performing a sport or activity to the best of your ability. Visualize yourself crossing the finish line in record time or sinking a fifteen-foot tournament-winning putt. See your success to the point that you can almost feel it. This is a great motivational meditation.

MANTRA

Use a mantra (phrase or sentence) or counting system to stimulate a meditative state. Repeat "I am strong, I am healthy," or any other mantra that inspires you, in your mind. Simple affirmations and mantras can fit almost any of your needs, from health and prosperity to relationships and creativity.

COUNT

In order to incorporate meditation into your run or jog, count your breath as you step. Repeatedly inhale for 6 steps and exhale for 6 steps. If you notice your mind wandering, simply acknowledge any exterior thoughts and put them aside for later. Eventually, you will have the ability to get out of your body and activate your mind, achieving a mind-body connection.

Jamie Lee Curtis's Meditation Teacher

When asked what she does to destress, Jamie Lee Curtis responded with one very enthusiastic word, "Meditate!" This actress, with more than fifty film and television credits under her belt, began her meditation practice four years ago. As she tells it, "I asked a meditation teacher, Ann Buck, to teach me how." Ann Buck considers herself "a spiritual friend" and is committed to helping people find their own teachers within themselves. She is sought after by thousands around the world and is even able to teach clients how to meditate over the phone. She explains, "I practice insight meditation [Vipassana], a simple and direct practice of moment-to-moment observation of the mind-body process through calm and focused awareness."

Vipassana is extremely useful for stress reduction as it offers the body mechanisms for dealing with stress. When teaching clients over the phone, Ann first establishes a customized basic meditation practice to untangle body, mind, and spirit. Guided meditations help unravel accumulated stresses and frustrations in an attempt to settle eventually into a loving and accepting state of being. Even if you can sit on a cushion for thirty minutes just a few times a week, practicing some form of concentration, you will find that you become more aware of your daily habits, energy, and presence, and you will feel a relaxing release. But this doesn't necessarily come naturally. You have to train your body and mind to go to that meditative space. Eventually, this training will sink deep into the recesses of your psyche and body, and your life will be positively affected.

Training takes time and commitment, both of which may be accelerated through the guidance of experts. So enroll in a class, inquire about a

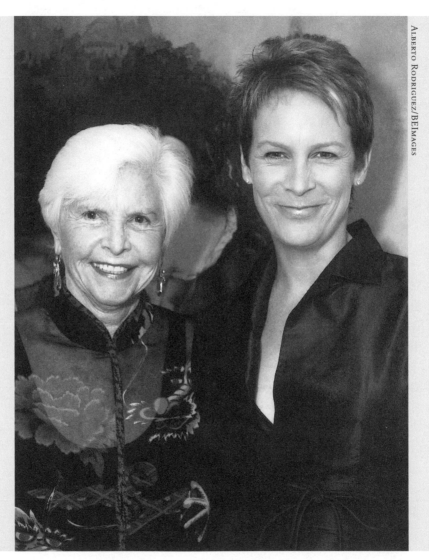

Jamie Lee Curtis and meditation teacher, Ann Buck.

Ann Buck's Recipe for Getting Started in Meditation

Begin with 10 minutes each day; eventually progress to 20 minutes.

Consistency is key. You must decide how much time you can dedicate each day to your practice. While the time that you allot for yourself may gradually increase, the important thing is to notice the changes in your life and self.

Allow yourself to reach a state of deep relaxation and let go.

meditation guru, or read books on meditation. "If you can't go to a center," Ann suggests, "get Sounds True—a catalog of spiritual tapes. Get beginning meditation tapes by Joseph Goldstein, Jack Kornfield, Shinzen Young, or Sharon Salzberg. People need to make a decision on what type of meditation [they are interested in practicing]. Do the research and find out what you are comfortable with."

Though many of her clients are celebrities who are extremely eloquent on film, when speaking about Ann, even her most articulate clients seem to fumble for words. The impact that Ann has had on countless lives and spirits transcends language. Celebrities, including Jamie, seek out her expertise for many reasons. Buck states, "I think many of us have found that fame and fortune isn't necessarily the answer [to happiness] and can [actually] contain a great deal of emptiness." Meditation can help you find yourself amid the chaos of everyday life. In a time when many of us grapple with self-judgment, insecurity, frustration, expectation, and anxiety, Ann teaches the essential tools that allow us to release our inner strife and lead longer, healthier, and happier lives. For Ann, meditation provides "the instant relief of being enough right now, just as I am."

Catherine Hicks on Rosary Beads and Prayer

Having grown up Catholic, Catherine Hicks, one of the stars of the WB hit *7th Heaven,* has spent many quiet hours in prayer. She has adopted her own regimen, using rosary beads "when the Spirit moves me." Akin to meditation, Catherine's near daily practice offers her a chance to take a breath, slow down, and reflect.

Amber Valletta's Morning and Night Ritual

Many of us may find it difficult to portion out a period within our jam-packed days to dedicate to ourselves. This is the exact reason that I often spend my "me-time" in the morning, before my day has really begun. The supermodel Amber Valletta does too. She tries to pray or meditate for a few minutes first thing in the morning and at night just before she falls asleep. She explains, "Meditating is a great way to start and end my day. I take a few deep breaths and make a vow to myself to be kind to people and have a good day. I thank the universe for my good blessings and then begin or end my day." This ritual has become regular for Amber. It is her way to be sure that she includes at least a few moments of "me-time" in every day.

The Art of Being Still

Though he is a renowned meditation expert and Zen Buddhist priest with more than a decade of training with Taizan Maezumi Roshi at the Zen Center of Los Angeles, has a book entitled *Zen Meditation in Plain English,* and runs a successful private psychotherapy and psychoanalytic practice in Santa Monica, John Daishin Buksbazen doesn't consider himself a guru. He says, "I am still a student because I remain open to a continuing and deepening realization about what our life really is." Well, if not a guru, he is, for certain, a teacher—one who offers a rare step-by-step introduction to the fundamentals and mechanics of meditating. And, as he says, there is no substitute for a good teacher. His book is the perfect guide for a beginner because it is easy to understand and clearly explains the principles of Zen meditation, which emphasizes breathing and sitting.

John practices the art of being still. He explains, "Many say Zen Buddhism is a religion, a philosophy, or a way of life. To me, Zen meditation is the practice of being still with clarity. Although it involves being still, it isn't static. Essential to Zen practice is the seated meditation called *zazen,* or sitting." Sometimes we find that our internal world of sensations, memories, hopes, and fears influences our ability to cope with the outer world. We may fall victim to mental and physical fatigue, which can eventually lead to the loss of our true selves. Zazen helps us reclaim our selves and restore the peace within us. "The next element is repetitious breathing." John goes on to explain that "the root for the words *spirit* and *breathe* is the same. To breathe in is to inspire, and to breathe out is to expire."

The beauty of meditation is its ability to quiet the mind. Zen meditation helps us find a mental breath. It teaches us how to sit actively still. We are not shutting off our brains. Rather, we are quieting the noise that clutters our minds and hinders clear thoughts. When our minds are cleared of excessive noise, we have a greater capability to think rationally. This mental and physical break also brings clarity and insight into our daily lives. Zen meditation is empowering yet brings a serene state of balance in which day-to-day worries seem inconsequential.

It is no wonder that celebrities are drawn to meditation, and John is no stranger to celebrity sightings. He says, "Celebrities are under extraordinary pressure to be centered. They want something to ground them. Meditation reintroduces us to a natural balance that we can then reinforce. It replenishes [celebrities'] sense of balance and sanity. It brings them to a quieter aspect of their inner life." For those who are already introspective and in tune with their inner selves, meditation is a way of connecting to others as well as the surrounding environment. John believes that "through meditation, the ability to observe and take in information is amplified. The senses are awakened, inspiring compassion. With heightened sympathy, we are better able to understand the perspectives of others. Understanding is a remedy for intolerance."

When we start a sport or practice, the first thing that many of us do is buy a new outfit and gear up. When I (Laurel) recently decided to take up tennis, I immediately headed for the sporting equipment store and walked out clad in a brand-new tennis skirt and visor with a perfectly strung racket in hand. I was ready for my new commitment to tennis. With meditation, though there isn't a required get-up, you can certainly enhance your practice by creating the proper mood. Creating a space, or simply buying a special candle, is the perfect way to begin a new practice.

John Daishin Buksbazen's Recipe for Getting Started in Meditation

Simply set aside some "quiet time."

Sit and breathe. To breathe is to inspire (to breathe in) and to expire (to breathe out). These words have the same root as *spirit*. Through the practice of conscious breathing, people may find their own spirituality.

Make your meditation practice a priority that you consistently incorporate into your day, at or near the same time each day.

Begin practicing for a short time (5 to 10 minutes), gradually increasing until you can sit for 20 minutes at a time.

Keep a few basic tips in mind—proper posture, breathing, and attention:

POSTURE

Seat yourself on the forward third of your chair, using a cushion if needed, so that your hips are a little higher than your knees.

Tilt your hips slightly by gently sliding the small of your back forward.

Extend your spine so that you are upright, and not leaning to either side or to the front or back.

Tuck in your chin slightly, and make sure your nose is over your navel and your ears aligned with your shoulders.

Place your left hand, palm up, on top of your right palm. Rest your hands in your lap, on top of your thighs.

Keep your eyes slightly open, looking downward to a point a few feet in front of you. Let them drift out of focus.

BREATHING

To begin, take a couple of deep, slow breaths through the mouth, and exhale freely.

Close your lips and swallow any saliva in your mouth.

Now breathe through your nose.

Place the tip of your tongue on the roof of your mouth just behind the front teeth.

Let each exhalation be relatively slow and deep, but avoid forced breathing. Your breathing will gradually slow and deepen by itself because of your posture and mental state.

Use your lower abdominal muscles to move air in and out of your body. As your abdomen expands, inhale as if filling an imaginary balloon in your lower belly. As you exhale, your abdomen naturally contracts, deflating this imaginary balloon.

Let your breathing become regular and continuous without holding your breath, straining, or gasping. Easy does it. No rush.

ATTENTION

Be aware of the sensations of your breath leaving and entering your body with each exhalation and inhalation.

Direct each breath into the center of your lower abdomen, about 2 or 3 inches below the navel.

As you exhale, silently count "one," continuing this number through the following inhalation.

At the next exhalation, count "two" silently, and so on, repeating the process of counting each exhale-inhale cycle as one breath.

When you have counted ten breath cycles, return to one and begin again. As an alternative to counting, closely follow the physical experience of breathing with all your attention.

If you notice your attention has wandered, or if you forget or lose count or go beyond ten, simply begin over again at one.

Let your attention remain with your breath. Be patient with yourself; it may take some time before you can fix your attention for an extended period of time.

If you find your mind becoming active with thoughts, memories, or emotions, allow yourself to acknowledge this and then return your attention to your breathing.

Goldie Hawn's Meditation Atrium

The überactress Goldie Hawn is also a meditation buff. According to a 2003 *New York Times* article, Goldie, a practicing Buddhist, has transformed the atrium of her Vancouver home into a meditation room. Sunlight floods the window-filled space, illuminating each of Goldie's inspired treasures. Silk pillows adorn the floor, beautiful potted plants fill the air with healthy oxygen, and statues of Buddha bejewel this sacred space. This is Goldie's personal meditation sanctuary, where she finds harmony even in the midst of madness.

Shannon Elizabeth's Grounding Meditation

"People used to tell me that I wasn't grounded enough; they don't say that anymore." Shannon Elizabeth practices a grounding meditation several times a week in order to feel more connected with the earth, with her rela-

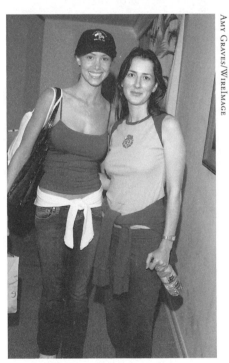

AMY GRAVES/WIREIMAGE

tionships, and with herself. After playing Nadia, the voluptuous exchange student in *American Pie* and *American Pie 2,* and sexy roles in *Jay and Silent Bob Strike Back* and *Scary Movie,* meditation allows Shannon to get back to herself and her spiritual roots.

"I am not a religious person, but I am a spiritual person," she reveals. "I believe that people around you have their own energies, and when they come into contact with your energies, some of theirs can be left behind. Sometimes you need to cleanse your space. To ground myself, I imagine that I have a tree trunk growing down my spine and into the core of the earth. After a while, the trunk is tainted with lingering energies from other people's presence. So I mentally blow up my old trunk and rebuild it, from my spine to the core of the earth. When I walk, I picture each step grounded to the earth. I imagine a white light from above coming down to surround and protect me. I do the same thing when I fly. The light protects the plane and the people around me. This is just something that works for me."

Shannon Elizabeth and Anna Getty.

Marla Maples's Kabbalah Meditations

Having lived a fast-paced, well-heeled, highly publicized life on the arm of one of New York's most infamous moneymen, Marla Maples certainly knows the importance of downtime. Now immersed in the more relaxed Southern California lifestyle, Marla has allowed her spiritual self to blossom. She explains, "I study Kabbalah, which I find to be an amazing practice that helps to take me out of the physical and into another dimension. Kabbalah helps me to see beyond the physical chaos and step into a more conscious realm. It helps me to draw more light into every situation." Though I (Laurel) am sure that the life she leads is extremely harried (flying around the world to fabulous functions, fighting traffic to and from film sets, and being chased by paparazzi), Marla's voice was one of the more serene that I have had the pleasure to hear. "I just meditated!" she disclosed. "I wanted to be in a more balanced state of mind when we spoke." In fact, she meditates every day, morning and night, for twenty minutes.

In order to combat the road rage caused by bumper-to-bumper traffic on the L.A. freeways, Marla practices destressing driving meditations. She says, "I try to get myself into a peaceful place and state of mind." While other drivers may be cursing the world and swearing up a storm, Marla simply goes with the flow, slow as it may be, until she arrives at her destination.

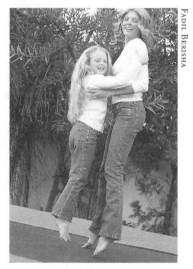

FADIL BERISHA

Marla Maples jumping on a trampoline with her daughter, Tiffany.

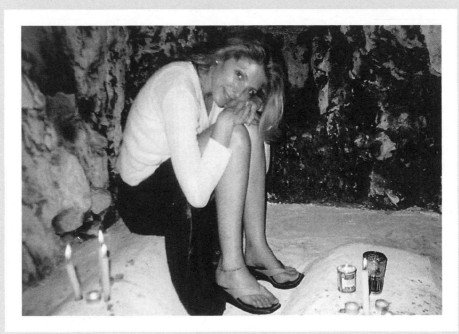

Marla just after meditating in the cave in the Upper Galilee where the Zohar was revealed to
Rabbi Shimon Bar'Yochai approximately two thousand years ago.

"In studying ourselves, we find the harmony that is our total existence. We do not make harmony. We do not achieve it or gain it. It is there all the time. Here we are, in the midst of this perfect way, and our practice is simply to realize it and then to actualize it in our everyday life." —Taizan Maezumi Roshi

RESOURCES

Vipassana Support Institute: (866) 666–0874

www.soundstrue.com

www.shinzen.org

Buddha's Little Instruction Book by Jack Kornfield

Zen Meditation in Plain English by John Daishin Buksbazen

www.zenmind.com

www.ladharma.com

Seeds of Consciousness, Affirmations for Daily Living, by Louise-Diana
    (see www.devross.com)

www.kabbalah.com

www.spiritualityforkids.com

Chapter Seven

Joyful Cooking

I grew up associating food with comfort.
—*Jenna von Oy*

IN TIMES of stress, many of us immediately turn to our comfort foods to lighten the load. This actually makes scientific sense since carbohydrates, fat, and chocolate in particular contain substances that unleash calm-provoking chemicals like serotonin and endorphins in our bodies. Unfortunately, the comfort food high lasts for just minutes. And after we binge, we are likely to stare at the mirror in self-disgust wracked with guilt. What comes out of guilt? More stress. And so the vicious cycle begins! While indulging once in a while is certainly healthy, going on a binge is not. If you really want the chocolate chip cookie, go for it. Just don't eat the entire bag. You can relieve stress without packing in countless grams of fat. In fact, the act of cooking itself can be relaxing.

Stress relieving as it may be, I (Laurel) never thought that I would be caught dead in the kitchen. I am a working woman who helps provide financially and emotionally for my family. The home-cooked meal, the wife who greets her husband returning from work in an apron with her hair perfectly pulled back, with a chicken roasting in the oven and vegetables on the stove (you know, the whole scene) evoked a sense of the 1950s housewife that I never wanted to become. Then, one night, as kind of a joke, I greeted my husband at the door wearing an adorable little apron that I bought in Portofino, Italy, playing the whole housewife role of taking off his shoes, handing him a drink, asking about his day, and finally serving a home-cooked meal that I had slaved for hours to create. It suddenly dawned on me that I love to cook (minus the other 1950s aspects)! After all those years of dismissing the idea of laying a finger on a frying pan for fear that I would become the stereotypical subservient wife, whose sole goal in life is to make her husband happy, I realized that I actually enjoy cooking, not just creating a great meal for my husband but for myself and my serenity. Cooking quickly became my method of destressing after a long day of work. The smile on my husband's face each night when he opens the door to a warm home filled with the smells of dinner, I must say, makes the whole experience even better.

Cooking can be relaxing and restorative; it needn't always be about feeding the family. Following a recipe, perhaps adding a new twist, making something up, or trying to interpret a favorite dish from a restaurant, each has its own creative and personal potential. Why else would *The Joy of Cooking* be a bestseller for generations? Even celebrities find time to cook. The supermodel Cindy Crawford and her husband, Rande Gerber, like to entertain at their home with friends and family. Both share the culinary duties, with Cindy stating, "I make a great shiksa brisket" (*Elle Decor*, November 2002).

Dr. James Rouse on Healing Through Food

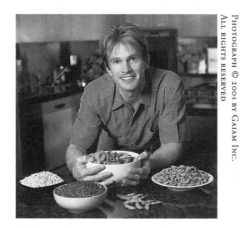

Dr. James Rouse

Dr. James Rouse, a naturopathic doctor and host of various wellness news segments for NBC, is a strong believer in the healing qualities of food. He explains, "Any time that we are utilizing and handling pleasant-smelling foods, we are encouraging the sense of smell. Smell is connected with the part of the brain that connects and partially controls our stress and pleasure. When we are handling and working with food, we are able to experience food on many levels . . . olfactorily, tactilely, and visually. The act of giving has also been shown to enhance our well-being as we are fostering a connection to self-care and love while connecting with and loving others. Simultaneously, food supports immune function. When we are relaxed in the kitchen, we encourage a hormonal 'expression' that supports a healthy mood, enhanced energy, and centeredness." Basically, almost every facet of food is pleasure promoting. Well, except maybe doing the dishes!

The act of cooking can certainly be relaxing. But in addition to the act itself, certain foods can directly affect mood and create feelings of calm. Dr. James (as he is called by patients) believes that particular foods help while others hinder our management of stress. Foods that are high in vitamins C, B_5, and B_6, as well as key minerals such as calcium, magnesium, and zinc, are essential in the production of stress-reducing hormones in the adrenal glands. Explains Dr. James, "These nutrients serve to support healthy hormone building blocks and enhance a healthy response to stress. Lean proteins are rich in the amino acid tryptophan, which, when combined with a complex carbohydrate, will support healthy levels of the relaxing and balancing brain chemical serotonin."

Dr. James's List of Stress-Management Foods

FRUITS

Apples	Flavonoids, fiber, quercetin
Bananas	Tryptophan, potassium
Blueberries	Antioxidants
Cherries	Melatonin, perillyl
Grapefruit	Vitamin C, pectin, dietary fiber
Lemons	Vitamin C, potassium
Oranges	Vitamin C, flavonoids
Strawberries	Ellagic acid (an antioxidant)

VEGETABLES

Arame seaweed Minerals, B vitamins, lignates
Broccoli Antioxidants, carotenoids, folate, calcium, indoles
Cabbage   Vitamin C, folate, glutamine (an amino acid)
Carrots Beta-carotene
Kale   Vitamin C, calcium
Mixed greens   Phytochemicals
Shiitake mushrooms   Immune support, vitamin D

NUTS AND SEEDS

Almonds   Lower cholesterol, healthy monosaturated fat,
                 protein, fiber
Basmati rice   Insoluble fiber, manganese
Hazelnuts   Omega-3 fatty acids
Lentils   Folate, magnesium, fiber
Oats   Fiber, magnesium, B vitamins, tryptophan
Pumpkin seeds   Zinc, magnesium
Whole wheat   Fiber, vitamin E, zinc, folate

PROTEIN AND DAIRY

Chicken, turkey   Tryptophan, protein
Cottage cheese   Calcium, protein, digestive cultures
Cow's milk   Tryptophan, calcium
Eggs   Omega-3 fatty acids, tryptophan

Fish   Omega-3 fatty acids, tryptophan, protein
Soybeans, soy milk   Calcium, protein, monounsaturated fats
String cheese   Calcium, protein, tryptophan
Tofu and tempeh Calcium, protein, monounsaturated fats
Yogurt   Calcium, tryptophan, acidophilus and bifidus

OILS

Canola oil   Omega-3 fatty acids, monounsaturated fats
Flaxseed oil   Omega-3 fatty acids, monounsaturated fats
Olive oil Omega-3 fatty acids, monounsaturated fats

HERBS

Chamomile, melissa   (Lemon balm)
Humulus   (Hops)
Passiflora   (Passionflower)
Reishi mushroom
Scutellaria   (Skullcap)
Valerian

SUPPLEMENTS AND TREATMENTS

B vitamins (especially B_3, B_5, B_6)
Calcium
Magnesium
Multivitamins, minerals

Pantothenic acid

Vitamin C

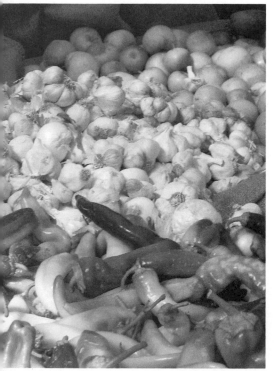

While certain foods are known to reduce stress and generate smiles, others may actually diminish the body's ability to handle stress. Unfortunately, many are daily components to the average person's diet. Obviously, we are not telling you to completely deny yourself the following tasty treats. Just try to remember that moderation is key when it comes to caffeine, chocolate, alcohol, ice cream, candy, cookies, chips, diet aids, fast foods, processed foods, refined sugars, soda, and white bread. If you are not ready to moderate your consumption of these dietary items, at the very least try to pair them with a healthy side dish—a piece of fruit with your breakfast croissant, a salad filled with lots of colors (carrots, peppers, dark greens, or corn) with your pizza lunch, or a fruit salad sprinkled with a dash of sugar as dessert after dinner. Even little things make a difference.

An Afternoon at a Farmers' Market

Cooking can include expeditions to local farmers' markets. Celebrities such as the *Six Feet Under* actress Rachel Griffiths, Edward Albert, and Ray Manzarek of The Doors have been seen spending leisurely weekend mornings at the Los Angeles area farmers' markets, sampling organic produce, learning about unusual vegetables, and watching cook-offs such as the

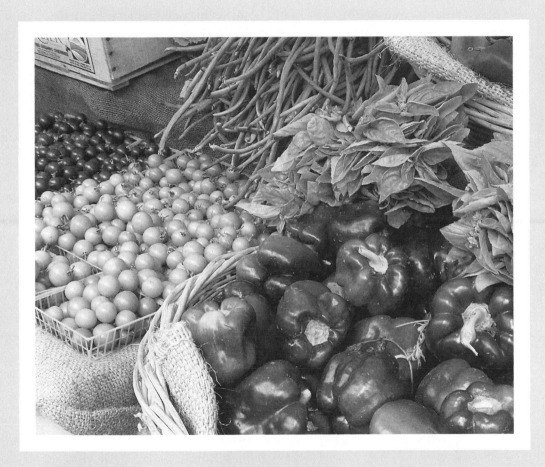

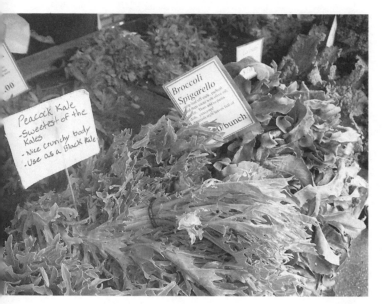

annual "Chili Cookoff" in Beverly Hills. For many, these trips are essential destressing elements in their weekend festivities. The scarlet, umber, gold, and green hues of seasonal apples and the aroma of turmeric at the local Indian stand provide a temporary respite.

The bright colors, sweet and sour smells, fruit and vegetable samplings, local bands, and social interaction make farmers' markets true feasts for the senses. Once you have selected the freshest broccoli, perfectly ripe strawberries, crunchy apples, and fragrant flowers, you stroll over to the always friendly mushroom man, who oftentimes throws in a few extra shiitake free of charge. The woman selling creamy homemade hand lotions always offers up a soothing sample, even if you aren't purchasing her wares today. You wave hello to your neighbor and your daughter's schoolteacher as an A-list celebrity, clad in a baseball cap and jeans, casually passes by. Suddenly, food is a social event, and we haven't even started cooking yet! But believe me, cooking with fresh fruits and vegetables, picked only hours, or at most days before, makes all the difference in the world.

Food can also elicit thoughts of distant

lands. Whether it is Italian pasta primavera with succulent tomatoes and extra-virgin olive oil, mouth-watering yellow Indian tandoori, or El Salvadoran tamales bursting with flavors, food evokes images, feelings, memories, and desires of traveling to exotic or very real places. Sometimes, the scent of a certain spice will induce you to recall moments more clearly than a photograph. Who knew that food was such a powerful thing?

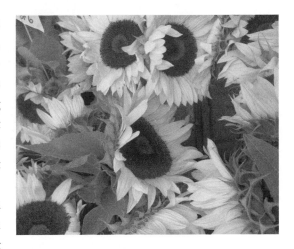

Trying to interpret a recipe remembered from a favorite vacation spot will transport you in time, in itself a relaxing retreat. I (Laurel) remember eating apple-crusted salmon at a tiny, off-the-beaten-path restaurant called El Pintor in Spain. It was quite a peculiar restaurant on a narrow little street that seemed as though it was plucked from a movie. We sat upstairs and were served by this unbelievably charismatic and friendly waiter, who stumbled over his English as we attempted to spew out a few words of Spanish. I honestly don't remember a time my family was happier. We laughed, told stories, and gorged ourselves on savory Spanish dishes. We went back three nights in a row, and each time I had that same salmon entrée.

The cookbook sections of your local bookstores, and even some supermarkets, are crammed with recipes that can fill your kitchen with the scent of Tuscany or Paris. The mere act of browsing is guaranteed to transport you, as cookbooks are often filled with photographs and personal stories of food adventures around the world.

If you are not quite ready to throw on an apron and get cookin', at least not without a little laying of the ground rules first, find a cooking class

Sharon's Farmers' Market Chunky Applesauce

MAKES 2 GENEROUS PORTIONS

Pare, core, and slice 4 medium apples.
  Combine:

  1 cup water
  ¼ cup sugar
  Dash mace

Bring to a boil.
  Add apple, cover, and simmer till tender (approximately 8 minutes).
  Cinnamon sticks can be added for flavor or garnish, and for the holidays add some tiny cinnamon candies.

that will teach you the fundamentals. Cooking classes offered at colleges, restaurants, markets, and specialty stores are a great way to discover the joy and relaxing benefits of cooking. Many are listed in local newspapers and range from the basics to esoteric offerings such as regional recipes, chocolate, sauces, sushi, and the Intermediate Knife Skills class through the Sur La Table Culinary Programs. Whole Foods Markets, the nation's leading organic and natural foods markets, offer cooking classes all year round. From "raw foods" to "Thanksgiving side dishes," these one-day programs are economical and informative.

If you are still not ready to start on your own cooking exploration, you

Laurel's Salmon and Apples (in Memory of Spain)

MAKES 2 SERVINGS

Preheat broiler.

1 apple, sliced thin
2 salmon fillets (each about 1½ inches thick)

Combine:

¼ cup cream
1 tablespoon brown sugar, plus extra for sprinkling
½ cup apple juice

Place cut apples on flesh side of salmon.

Line a cake pan with aluminum foil.

Place salmon on foil, skin side down.

Pour liquid mixture over top.

Sprinkle with brown sugar.

Broil fish until glaze begins to blister and brown, about 3 minutes.

Cover fish loosely with foil. Cinnamon sticks can be added for flavor or garnish.

Broil until fish is cooked through (about 5 minutes longer).

Transfer fish to plates.

Enjoy!

can at least begin to utilize food for its smile-producing effects by eating healthfully. For many of you, healthy food may still be a foreign language, so how about if we tempt your taste buds with a few mind-mending massages in addition to the health food? One way to make a jump start into the healthy food world is a visit to a spa.

Conscious Cooking with Cary Neff

The central element of spa resorts is providing guests with world-class tools of relaxation and comfort, in the hope that these tools will immediately add benefit to their lives and continue to be of assistance to them when they return to their regular lives. Many of us find refuge at a spa for more than the treatments. The chef Cary Neff is often a major reason that celebrities choose a specific spa resort for a renewing getaway. Cary is the head chef at La Costa—one of California's most celebrated spa resorts. Before his arrival at La Costa, Cary spent several years as the head chef of Miraval Life in Balance resort and spa in Arizona. His goal is "to teach guests new habits of enjoying balanced nutrition through making conscious decisions in regard to the food they purchase, prepare, and eat."

Food is a fundamental element at spa resorts because it has the power to unify. The head chef may utilize indigenous ingredients prepared in a low-fat, no-fat, vegetarian, vegan, raw, organic, or indulgent fashion, setting the ground rules for the overall experience. Cary's personal taste, and the taste he implements at each of his resorts, is conscious cuisine. While spas are often identified as promoting a low-fat lifestyle, Cary doesn't necessarily follow that rule. Instead, he believes in food awareness and the use of the best ingredients available. In lieu of butter, Cary is able to achieve great taste with healthy olive oil or chicken or vegetable stock. When fresh organic fruits and vegetables are available, they are his choice. When fish is flown in from the best fish markets throughout the United States or Europe, you will probably find it on your plate a few hours later. While health consciousness is a central ingredient to Cary's cooking, he also has respect for the occasional indulgence. But instead of cheap chocolate, he uses the best and richest available, making it less necessary to devour the entire dessert because your palate will be overwhelmed by the taste after just a few bites.

"Other than the air we breathe, food is the most essential element in our lives," says Cary. While each culture of the world uses food for nourishment, many have elevated its importance in other aspects of life. Food is used as currency or for trade. Food is also used to celebrate festive occasions, such as weddings, commencements, holiday gatherings, birthdays, and funerals. "The simple act of eating not only provides our bodies with daily nourishment but provides comfort, enjoyment, satisfaction, and sensual pleasure to our lives. When we embrace a more conscious approach to eating, life gets better."

While food is used to fulfill a physical need, in times of celebration and for social occasions it can also be used to satisfy emotional needs. Food can be a vehicle to destress. Relax and enjoy the healthy, well-made meal or take pleasure in the company of friends and family while savoring a delectable treat.

Once you have selected the scrumptious ingredients for your meal, Cary suggests that you "grant yourself artistic freedom to use the vibrant colors of the food you prepare to make your meal look exquisitely good for you—even if it's just for you, and even if it's only a sandwich and fruit. Women often work hard to make everything perfect and pretty for others but fail to treat themselves in the same manner. Be the master chef of *your meals.*"

Try to prepare your food "consciously." That is, make an effort to select and prepare healthy foods. *Healthy* doesn't necessarily mean tasteless; it simply means paying careful attention to the choices you make. Cary creates delicious conscious cuisine that is loved by calorie counters and ravenous carnivores alike. He makes "conscious efforts to eliminate or reduce

Cary's Recipe for Happy Shopping

Take the chore out of shopping for food.

Purchase toiletries, household items, and nonperishable items in bulk, separate from food shopping. Do this type of necessity shopping once or twice a month.

On a daily or weekly basis, seek out markets that provide high-quality seasonal produce that's at its peak of ripeness and flavor.

Choose high-quality meats, poultries, and seafood.

Slow down! Stroll through the produce aisles and breathe in the fresh scent of vibrant in-season fruits and vegetables. Allow the freshness of the available produce, rather than the choice of meat, guide you in your meal planning. For instance, if the berries or wild mushrooms look and smell fantastic, buy them, regardless of whether you are cooking steak, chicken, fish, or tofu. Take them home and have fun re-creating classic dishes.

Cooking will be more like play than a chore!

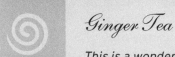

Ginger Tea

MAKES 5 SERVINGS

This is a wonderful way to start each day with a cleaning pick-me-up!

½ cup ginger juice (you can use a juicer, or grate the ginger, place the grated
ginger in a piece of cheesecloth, and squeeze out the juice)
⅓ cup honey
½ lemon, squeezed
5 cups spring water

Combine ingredients. After squeezing the juice out of it, toss the lemon into the water. Bring to a boil; simmer for 15 to 20 minutes. Remove lemon and serve.

PER SERVING:

CALORIES: 60; FAT: 0 GRAMS

excessive amounts of fats and calories, which is far different than seeking to eat fat-free and low-calorie foods." He says, "I don't count calories (and neither should you). Instead, pay attention and count the food types that you eat and maintain appropriate portion sizes. Choose whole grain and complex carbohydrates rather than highly processed foods. And always choose to eat a balanced meal in nutritional value and portion. You will immediately notice the difference in how you feel at work and play. When you begin to eat consciously or mindfully, life gets better. You will start to notice the wonderful flavor of a luscious tomato or juicy peach or the dissatisfaction of a mealy apple. Make satisfying decisions on your next purchase of a tomato or a peach, and understand the texture of a mushy apple."

But by all means do not give up on your favorite indulgent foods. There is such a thing as a healthy indulgence. If you crave a cookie, have one. If that coffee ice cream is calling your name, scoop some up. Just determine the appropriate stopping point, and be sure to stop there. Your taste buds and your craving will be satisfied.

Spinach and Strawberry Salad with Honey Dijon Vinaigrette

MAKES 8 CUPS

SERVING SIZE: 1 CUP

PRESENTED BY MIRAVAL LIFE IN BALANCE

Contrasting tastes, textures, and colors make this dish a feast for the senses. Add grilled chicken, pork, veggie burger, tofu, or shrimp to make a dynamite main course.

6 cups cleaned, trimmed, and dried spinach (packed)

1½ cups sliced strawberries (slices about ¼-inch thick)

1 tablespoon toasted sunflower seeds

1 small red onion, thinly sliced

1 tablespoon rice vinegar

2 tablespoons honey

2 teaspoons Dijon mustard

Salt and pepper to taste

1 head radicchio, cored, washed, and leaves separated

⅓ cup enoki mushrooms

Tear spinach into bite-size pieces and place in a salad bowl. Add strawberries, sunflower seeds, and onion. In separate bowl, whisk together vinegar, honey, mustard, salt and pepper. Pour the dressing over the spinach and toss lightly. Place one radicchio leaf on each plate. Arrange the spinach in each radicchio cup. Garnish with enoki mushrooms. PER SERVING: CALORIES: 50; FAT: 1 GRAM

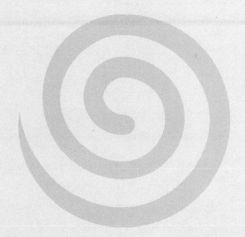

Beet Couscous and Steamed Organic Baby Vegetables with Pan-Seared Orange Roughy and Lemon Garlic Sauce

MAKES 4 SERVINGS

PRESENTED BY MIRAVAL LIFE IN BALANCE

- ¼ teaspoon extra-virgin olive oil
- 4 4-ounce orange roughy fillets
- 2 tablespoons fresh mixed herbs
- ¼ teaspoon sea salt
- ⅛ teaspoon freshly ground black pepper
- 1 medium zucchini, julienned
- 1 medium yellow squash, julienned
- 1 medium carrot, julienned
- ¼ cup water
- ¼ cup white wine
- 2 cups beet couscous
- 1 cup lemon garlic sauce

Heat a large sauté pan over medium high heat and add olive oil to lightly coat the bottom of the pan. Season the orange roughy with the herbs, salt, and pepper. Add orange roughy to the pan and sear on one side for 2 minutes to brown. Turn over and sear the other side for 1 minute. Add the zucchini, yellow squash, and carrots in three bundles, with the water and wine. Cover and steam for 1 minute.

To plate: Arrange ½ cup of beet couscous on each plate. Place the vegetables on three sections of the plate, forming a triangle around the couscous. Top the couscous with the orange roughy, and drizzle 1 to 2 tablespoons of lemon garlic sauce over fish.

PER SERVING:
CALORIES: 350; PROTEIN: 25 GRAMS; TOTAL FAT: 2 GRAMS;
SATURATED FAT: 0 GRAMS; CARBOHYDRATES: 55 GRAMS; DIETARY FIBER: 5 GRAMS;
CHOLESTEROL: 25 MILLIGRAMS; SODIUM: 540 MILLIGRAMS

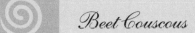

Beet Couscous

MAKES 10 SERVINGS

PRESENTED BY MIRAVAL LIFE IN BALANCE

Beet juice with the addition of cinnamon makes a deliciously sweet broth that adds vibrant color and great tasting nutrients to couscous.

¼ teaspoon extra-virgin olive oil
½ cup diced red onion
2 cups Israeli couscous
1 cup unsweetened apple juice
3 cups fresh beet juice (about 15 medium beets)
1 teaspoon ground cinnamon
½ teaspoon sea salt
¼ teaspoon ground white pepper

Heat a medium saucepan over medium high heat and add the olive oil to coat only the bottom of the pan. Stir in the onion and cook until just softened, about 2 minutes. Add the couscous, apple juice, beet juice, and seasonings. Mix well and bring to a boil. Reduce heat to a low simmer and cover the pan.

Steam the couscous for about 45 minutes or until the liquid is absorbed and the couscous is bright red.

PER ½ CUP:

CALORIES: 180; PROTEIN: 6 GRAMS; TOTAL FAT: 0 GRAMS;
SATURATED FAT: 0 GRAMS; CARBOHYDRATES: 38 GRAMS; DIETARY FIBER: 2 GRAMS;
CHOLESTEROL: 0 MILLIGRAMS; SODIUM: 260 MILLIGRAMS

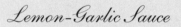

Lemon-Garlic Sauce

MAKES 3½ CUPS

PRESENTED BY MIRAVAL LIFE IN BALANCE

1 teaspoon extra-virgin olive oil
¾ cup minced fresh garlic
1 cup finely chopped green onions (about 1 bunch)
½ cup fresh lemon juice (juice of about 4 lemons)
¼ cup white wine
¼ cup chopped fresh thyme
¼ teaspoon freshly ground black pepper
1½ quarts vegetable stock
¼ teaspoon sea salt

¼ teaspoon honey

3 tablespoons cornstarch mixed with 4 tablespoons vegetable stock

Heat a saucepot over medium heat and add the olive oil to coat the bottom of the pot. Stir in the garlic and green onions, and cook until onions have softened, about 2 minutes. Stir in the lemon juice, wine, thyme, and pepper. Cook until the sauce is reduced and the pot is almost dry to concentrate the flavors. Add the stock and bring to a boil. Reduce heat and simmer for 15 minutes. Season with salt and honey.

Strain the onion mixture through a colander lined with cheesecloth or a fine mesh strainer.

Place the strained sauce back in the saucepot and bring to a low boil. Mix in the cornstarch mixture and cook, stirring constantly, until the sauce thickens and coats the back of a spoon. Use the sauce immediately or cool it down in an ice bath. Store in an airtight container for up to 1 week in the refrigerator or freeze for about 1 month.

PER ¼ CUP:
CALORIES: 60; PROTEIN: 1 GRAM; TOTAL FAT: 0 GRAMS;
SATURATED FAT: 0 GRAMS; CARBOHYDRATES: 12 GRAMS

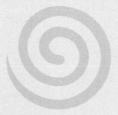

Warm Pineapple and Mango Tart

MAKES 6 SERVINGS

PRESENTED BY MIRAVAL LIFE IN BALANCE

Warm Pineapple and Mango Tart and Pineapple Upside-Down Cake are great-tasting desserts and the results of a conscious effort to eliminate or reduce excessive amounts of fats and calories.

FILLING

2 cups small diced pineapple

2 mangoes, peeled and cut into small pieces

4 tablespoons fruit sweet syrup or corn syrup

1 vanilla bean, split in half lengthwise, beans scraped out

CRUST

3 cups rolled oats

¼ cup fruit sweet syrup or corn syrup

Preheat the oven to 350°F (175°C).

For the filling: In a mixing bowl, combine the pineapple, mangoes, syrup, and vanilla bean. Set aside.

For the crust: In another mixing bowl, stir the oats and syrup. The oats should stick together when pressed with fingers.

Place 6 (4-inch) pastry rings on a baking sheet and spray with cooking spray. Or spray an 8-inch cake pan with cooking spray.

Using about 2 tablespoons of oats per ring, press into the rings to form a bottom crust. Spoon ½ cup of pineapple mixture into each ring and press down to remove any excess air. Sprinkle 2 tablespoons of oats on top of the pineapple to form the top crust.

If using a cake pan, press half the oats into the bottom of the pan. Pour pineapples on top. Press down to remove any excess air. Sprinkle the remaining oats on top of the pineapple to form the top crust.

Bake for 12 minutes or until oats are golden brown.

PER SERVING:

CALORIES: 270; PROTEIN: 7 GRAMS; TOTAL FAT: 3 GRAMS;

SATURATED FAT: 0.5 GRAMS; CARBOHYDRATES: 55 GRAMS;

DIETARY FIBER: 7 GRAMS; CHOLESTEROL: 0 GRAMS; SODIUM: 5 MILLIGRAMS

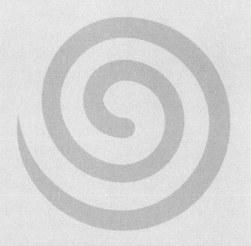

Pineapple Upside-Down Cake

MAKES 16 SERVINGS

PRESENTED BY MIRAVAL LIFE IN BALANCE

¼ cup honey

3 cups sliced pineapple

1 tablespoon unsalted butter

2 tablespoons prune puree

¾ cup raw cane sugar

1 egg

1 teaspoon vanilla extract

1½ cups unbleached all-purpose flour

1½ teaspoons baking powder

½ teaspoon baking soda

½ teaspoon ground cinnamon

¼ teaspoon sea salt

¾ cup low-fat buttermilk

Preheat the oven to 350°F (175°C). Heat the honey, and pour into a 10-inch sprayed cake pan. Arrange the pineapple slices spoke fashion, working from the center of the pan to the edge.

Cream together the butter, prune puree, and sugar with a mixer at medium speed for 4 minutes. Add egg and vanilla; beat well.

Combine the flour, baking powder, baking soda, cinnamon, and salt; stir well.

Alternating with the buttermilk, slowly add the flour mixture to the creamed mixture, beginning and ending with the flour mixture; mix well after each addition.

Spoon the batter evenly over the pineapple. Bake for 35 to 40 minutes or until a wooden pick inserted in the center comes out clean. Let cool in pan for 5 minutes. To serve, run a knife around the edge and turn the pan over on a serving plate.

PER SERVING:
CALORIES: 100; PROTEIN: 2 GRAMS; TOTAL FAT: 1 GRAM;
SATURATED FAT: 0.5 GRAMS; CARBOHYDRATES: 21 GRAMS;
DIETARY FIBER: LESS THAN 1 GRAM; CHOLESTEROL: 15 MILLIGRAMS; SODIUM: 115 MILLIGRAMS

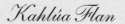

Kahlúa Flan

MAKES 9 SERVINGS

1¼ cups granulated sugar
½ cup water
1¼ cups fat-free milk
1½ cups 2 percent milk
½ cup half and half
2 cinnamon sticks
1 vanilla bean, split and scraped
6 large egg whites
1 large egg
⅓ cup evaporated raw cane sugar
1½ tablespoons Kahlúa
½ tablespoon molasses

Place the granulated sugar and water in a saucepan and cook over medium heat, stirring constantly until sugar is dissolved. Bring to a boil and cook until sugar turns amber. Remove from heat and pour into 9 lightly greased 4-ounce ramekins. Set aside.

Place the milks, half and half, cinnamon sticks, and vanilla bean in a saucepan and bring to a simmer over low heat. Remove from heat, cover, and steep for at least 30 minutes. Return pan to stove and bring the mixture back to a boil.

Meanwhile combine the egg whites, egg, cane sugar, Kahlúa, and molasses in a bowl. Whisk the egg mixture into the hot milk. Strain the mixture and pour into prepared ramekins. Bake in a water bath at 325°F for 1 hour or until set. Remove and chill.

To serve, run a hot knife around the inside edges of the ramekins and invert onto plates.

PER SERVING:
CALORIES: 160; PROTEIN: 6 GRAMS; TOTAL FAT: 2.4 GRAMS;
SATURATED FAT: 1.5 GRAMS; CARBOHYDRATES: 26 GRAMS; DIETARY FIBER: 0 GRAMS;
CHOLESTEROL: 35 MILLIGRAMS; SODIUM: 90 MILLIGRAMS

Catherine Hicks on Cooking

Catherine Hicks, star of the WB's *7th Heaven,* has been called "the Donna Reed of the new millennium." Because she plays the mother of seven children on the series that has been the WB's highest-rated program for the past seven seasons, many perceive her as a "supermom," adept at everything . . . including cooking. Not so, says Catherine, who feels a tinge of guilt for not being able to spend more time with her real-life daughter in the kitchen.

While growing up in Scottsdale, Arizona, Catherine spent time in the kitchen with her stay-at-home mother. This is an experience that she has tried to replicate for herself and her daughter, Katie. Even if it means getting up at 5:30, before she is due on the set, Catherine makes breakfast for her family every day. This is her "me-time," a time to conjure up the happy memories of her childhood and to create something warm and nutritious for her husband and daughter. Her daughter is often at her side as Catherine tries to create the experiences that will make the same memories Catherine holds so dear.

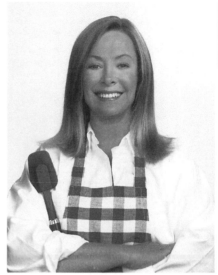

CATHERINE HICKS

Catherine Hicks in the kitchen.

Catherine doesn't like the rigidity of conforming to a recipe. "Chances are," says the actress, "I won't have one of the ingredients that the recipe calls for," so she has created her own simple solutions. One of her favorites is kugel.

Other "me-time" escapes for Catherine are local French restaurants, where her only companion is the *New York Times.* She loves the civility and small portions of French food; being a Francophile, Hicks just plain loves the "Frenchness" of the experience.

Since many of her best memories revolve around food and mealtime, Catherine teamed up with her girlfriends Cynthia Gould, Sandra Brinckerhoff, and Georgene Grattan, all adept in the kitchen, in a business venture called Easy Does It. This lunch box–style kit is filled with easy recipes, together with accompanying seasoning and sauce packages, designed to make meal preparation easy and stress free. The kit helps Catherine expand from her "usual repertoire of eight rotating dishes." And the packets are premeasured (no need to open eight spice jars or run to the neighbor's

Catherine's Kugel

YIELDS 4 SERVINGS

(All of the ingredients are approximate; to be specific would defeat the creative experience!)

YOU WILL NEED
   ½ stick of butter
   3 eggs
   1½ cups milk
   1 cup flour
   Raspberry jam
   Fresh whipped cream, not too stiff, sweetened with sugar

HOW TO
Put the butter in a brownie-size Pyrex pan.

   Melt the butter in the oven so that it is gently bubbling, at 400°F for 10 to 15 minutes.

   In a blender, place the eggs, milk, and flour. Blend 3 to 4 minutes, until frothy and airy.

   Add the blended ingredients to the hot pan and immediately return it to the oven.

   Bake another 30 minutes. You are making a giant popover; watch the pan so that your concoction doesn't get too dark.

   Remove the pan from the oven.

   Slice into wedges.

   Dollop or slather with jam and whipped cream.

Barbecue Chicken from Easy Does It

YOU WILL NEED

   1 2½–3-pound chicken cut in half
   3 packets Easy Does It BBQ Base (this is delicious and different because the
      ingredients include pears and apricots)
   1 packet Easy Does It Special Shake

HOW TO

Wash the chicken thoroughly.

   Preheat the oven to 350°F.

   Coat the chicken with BBQ Base, cover, and marinate at room temperature for at least 2 hours.

   Sprinkle with Special Shake.

   Place the chicken in a roasting pan.

   Add ¾ cup water and bake 45 minutes per side, basting every 15 minutes.

   Or, if you want to grill either in the broiler or on an outdoor barbecue, arrange the chicken on the grill or broiler pan. Using a low flame, cook, turning and basting frequently until browned on all sides (25 to 30 minutes per side). Broil about 6 inches from heat source, adding water to the pan if necessary.

for some esoteric spice you haven't stocked) to serve four, so that your family can finish the meal, or you single gals can have great leftovers. Says Catherine, "One of my favorites is the Barbecue Chicken, which I love because, finally, the family doesn't say, 'Chicken, . . . Again!?'"

Akasha's Fabulous Fare

Michael Jackson, Angelina Jolie, Barbra Streisand, Billy Bob Thornton, Pierce Brosnan and Keely Shaye Smith, and Kyle MacLachlan have all experienced the joys of Chef Akasha's prepared food. Her healthy and organic delights have been the talk of the upper-echelon Los Angeles crowd for years. In fact, some celebrities covet her food so much that they put her on staff and relish her fabulous fare morning, noon, and night whether they are at their Los Angeles, New York, or London homes, or traveling the world. Akasha is truly an in-demand chef. Because so many people, celebrities and noncelebs alike, vie for her attention, Akasha has become quite the successful caterer.

Though cooking, and talking about cooking (on television shows and in magazines), is Akasha's full-time career, she originally aspired to be an artist. Cooking was merely a hobby. Well, soon her hobby transformed into a job, and that job into a career, and now cooking is Akasha's life. More than one A-lister has thanked goodness that Akasha's artistic abilities proved to be more fruitful when it came to food than when it came to paint. She explains, "Most celebrities work real hard—sometimes getting up at 4:00 A.M., working fifteen- to seventeen-hour days. They just feel better when they eat healthy. They have more energy and endurance." Akasha is known for her fresh ingredients and flavorful food. She says, "My clients know that

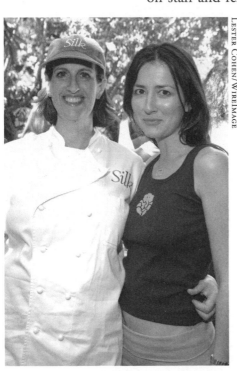

LESTER COHEN/WIREIMAGE

Chef Akasha and Anna Getty.

Akasha's Recipe for How to Begin

Watch the Food Network. Go to their Web site: www.foodnetwork.com.

Take a cooking class at Sur La Table, Whole Foods Market, a specialty market, or a restaurant. There are also cooking schools all over the United States.

Go to a bookstore and read cookbooks.

Two more of Akasha's favorite Web sites: FoodTV.com and Kitchenlink.com

cooking and eating healthy food is destressing. They know that I'm going out to the farmers' market to get the best-quality and healthiest produce."

Catering to the needs of her stressed-out clients, sometimes at odd times of the day and night, can wreak havoc on Akasha's adrenal system, too. She turns to food, healthy food, to destress. She explains, "When I'm stressed, I make cream of zucchini soup and wheat-free corn bread, which is quick and easy. Plus, it is comforting. Blended food is easier to digest. Just throw a bunch of zucchini into a food processor." Certain foods can also conjure up wonderful memories, perhaps of a simpler time. Akasha notes, "I find that people love to eat and make what their grandmothers make. It takes you to a different place."

Anna Getty's Food Gatherings

"There is a real ritual around eating," says Anna Getty. "I love the slow-food movement in Italy. Sometimes those lunches and dinners go on for

Anna's Recipe for a Connection over Food

It is very important to create the atmosphere.
   Invite a bunch of friends and family members over.
   Include the food preparation in the event.
   Ask your sister-in-law to chop the dill.
   Your best friend can create the marinade.

   Laugh.
   Drink wine.
   Tell stories.
   And finally eat.

Then enjoy more laughter, wine, and stories.

five hours." Food preparation can be an incredibly social yet simultaneously relaxing event. Everyone can stand around in the kitchen laughing, gossiping, drinking wine, and sampling the dishes. Anna recounts, "I love the whole process of tasting, adding spices, and experimenting with new recipes on whoever is here. Having your guests taste the different dishes as they come along is a great way of incorporating them into the meal. Sometimes I will cook for three days straight. That is what we did when my husband and I went to his hometown in Indiana for Thanksgiving. I researched recipes online before and found a great one for pumpkin cheesecake. I am a vegetarian, but I allow myself a treat once in a while."

After dinner, when everyone's stomach is full, "we sit around drinking our wine, talking, and laughing. Connecting through a meal is a very human response." Having everyone pitch in and enjoying a great meal together can give a sense of community that many big cities lack these days.

Constantly expanding her food knowledge, Anna turns to Chef Akasha for cooking class referrals and heads-ups on the newest vegetarian restaurants. Sometimes you need a break from three days of preparation followed by a five-hour meal!

Chef Elisa Gross's Nurture Through Nourishment

Food can be more than nourishment; it also has the ability to nurture and balance the body, mind and soul. Many of Elisa Gross's (of L'oven Life), clients are celebrities looking to transform their bodies in preparation for upcoming film and television roles. Elisa says, "I provide healthy comfort to people through the food that I make for them. The soothing energy, passion, and creativity that I put into the food, as well as the food itself, is important." As is believed in the ayurvedic tradition (one which Elisa studies), certain foods have properties that contribute to stress reduction. For example, romaine lettuce contains opiates, known for reducing stress, and asparagus is used medicinally as a nerve sedative. Ghee (clarified butter) cradles the nervous system and aids in the absorption of calming cooking herbs and spices, such as cardamom, coriander (cilantro), fennel, and cumin. How ingredients are combined, as well as texture, temperature, and taste (sweet, sour, salty, pungent, astringent, and bitter) are important factors in Ayurveda.

Elisa has worked to reshape and replenish the bodies of several well-known celebrities, including Thomas Jane as he prepared for *The Punisher*. His diet required constant adjustments and changing ratios of fats, carbohydrates, and protein in order to fulfill his weekly goals. Elisa prepared macrobiotic meals for Madonna and alkaline, blood-type specific, cleansing meals for David Duchovny. During David's cleanse, he admits that, "Each time, it was very important for me to undergo this delicate endeavor with as little disturbance to my daily routine as possible. Elisa made this available through her culinary expertise, her nutritional awareness, and her practical approch toward clean food." Pink also benefited from the cleanse and from Elisa's healthy ratio specific dietary regimen to compliment her workout.

Marla Maples—One Less Stressed Actress

Marla Maples is one of Elisa's clients. In fact, Marla, her boyfriend, and her mom treated themselves to Elisa's detoxifying cleanse. They were given eight ten ounce cups of water per day, several glasses of fruit and vegetable juices, and alkaline and detoxifying foods, such as quinoa, millet, almonds, walnuts, broccoli leafy greens, squash, green beans, carrots, apples, grapes, blueberries, and pears to promote cleansing of their systems. Elisa not only keeps the meals healthy, but her creative approach to holistic cuisine doesn't sacrifice any of the flavor. While Marla loves to cook for herself, especially with fresh, organic fruits and vegetables, she allowed Elisa to take charge of her family's cleanse (though Marla's daughter didn't participate). "I feel like we live in a toxic world, and I believe that during the spring and fall it is good to jump-start the system," says Marla. "A cleanse gives you a chance to get back in rhythm. Elisa just made life so simple and our bodies so clean." When not cleansing, Marla squeezes herself fresh ginger juice as a quick detox. It is believed that when the body is cleared of toxins, the mind follow. Marla explains, "I have a wheatgrass juicer and once a week I juice ginger instead of wheatgrass. It is a great way to cleanse the liver."

Jenna von Oy's Comforting Cooking

The actress Jenna von Oy chooses not to turn to a personal chef for her culinary needs. Instead, she enjoys cooking for herself. At twenty-seven years old, and with a successful acting career under her belt (she starred on *Blossom* for four and a half years and most recently played Stevie on *The Parkers*), Jenna has been working since the age of six. Though her work schedule was hectic, and quite unlike that of your average preteen, family remained integral to her life. Jenna's father, who was actually in the restaurant business, cooked up gourmet meals that enticed the entire family to gather around the table. "I grew up associating food with comfort," says Jenna. "I developed a process by keeping an eye on what my father was doing in the kitchen. Now I automatically know what herbs to use." Cooking continues to be therapeutic for Jenna. As her father did, she loves to cook for a bunch of people in the comfort of her home. "I'm not huge on following recipes. I prefer to re-create meals that I like at restaurants." Apparently, she is able to re-create a few of her own special dishes, because her friends have begun to request their favorites. She says, "My friend Dulé Hill (of *The West*

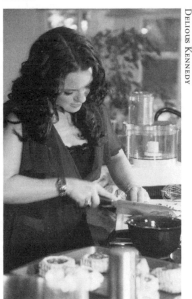

DELIOUS KENNEDY

Jenna von Oy cooking.

Jenna's "Tuscany Here We Come" Tart

YIELDS 6 SERVINGS ON 1 TART EACH

The sauce: This sauce should be prepared at least an hour before serving, as it needs time to cool in the refrigerator.

YOU WILL NEED

3 ripe tomatoes
¼ cup goat cheese
A pinch of salt
2 tablespoons olive oil

Boil the tomatoes in water and add a little salt until the skin begins to peel off (approximately 7 to 8 minutes).

Remove the tomatoes from the water and pull off the remaining skin.

Dice the tomatoes into chunks, removing the bases of the stems, and blend in a food processor.

Add just a bit of goat cheese, a pinch of salt, and olive oil.

Blend until smooth and refrigerate.

The tart: For this tart, I like to use Pepperidge Farm frozen puff pastries. They come in a package of six small tarts and each is the perfect serving size for one appetizer. They are also a quick and simple substitution for the frustration of attempting your own.

YOU WILL NEED

1 package of frozen puff pastries
2 Roma tomatoes, sliced
1 tablespoon goat cheese per tart
1–4 small sprigs fresh basil, julienned
Drizzle of olive oil
1 tablespoon melted butter

Place the puff pastries on an ungreased cookie sheet and bake at 400°F for 20 to 25 minutes. They will become slightly browned.

Gently lift the top off each pastry with a fork and put a slice of Roma tomato, a piece of goat cheese, and thinly sliced (julienned) basil inside.

Drizzle a very small amount of olive oil over these ingredients.

(Please note: These ingredients should not be overflowing. A small amount in each is sufficient.)

Replace the top of the pastry, and brush melted butter over each pastry. This will aid in browning.

Put the pastries back in the oven for 10 minutes.

The serving: I like to put each pastry in the center of a small plate. I pour a bit of sauce around each one and sprinkle fresh basil around as well. If you can find basil olive oil at your local supermarket, drizzle a bit of that on top for flavor.

Serve and enjoy!

Baked Apples

This is a sweet dessert, snack or breakfast that is widely used in Ayurvedic cooking and can also be used while cleansing. This is not only tasty, but aids in digestion as well.

4 apples
1 cup apple juice or water
4 large dates (remove pits)
$1/8$ cup raisins
$1/8$ cup chopped almonds
$1/8$ cup chopped walnuts
$1 1/2$ tablespoons cinnamon
$1/4$ teaspoon cardamom
$1/4$ teaspoon dry ginger or $1/2$ teaspoon fresh chopped ginger
2 teaspoons fresh lemon juice

Preheat oven to 375° degrees. Using an apple corer, remove the cores from the apples and put the apples in a baking dish. Mix all the ingredients except for the juice/water. Pack the mixture into the hollow center of the apples. Pour the liquid into the dish so it sits at the bottom ensuring the apples moisten while cooking. Cover and bake for 40 minutes to 1 hour, or until soft.

Though not specified in this recipe, it is always best to use organic ingredients whenever possible.

Wing) used to love my chicken cacciatore when he was a struggling actor. He still calls me up and asks if I happen to be making that dish. If I am, he will be 'right over.' "

While food with friends is great, Jenna also finds comfort in curling up with a good book and a good plate of food after a hard day on set. She explains, "After a stressful day, in order to destress, I would make a platter of French cheeses and olives." Sometimes, spurred on by the food, she reminisces about places she has traveled to, things she has seen, and experiences she has had. "Recently, I had lunch with a friend at a French restaurant. As the hours flew by, we reminisced about travel in Europe. The food helped evoke those memories." Jenna would love to go to cooking school or create a cookbook filled with recipes from family and friends, particularly from different cultures.

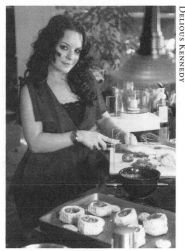

Jenna von Oy in the kitchen.

Tracee Ross Is "Queen of the Salad"

The *Girlfriends* star Tracee Ross loves to savor her "me-time" experiences with food. When she cooks for herself, she sets the table ("I have these great hot pink and green dishes that I love to use!"), turns down the lights, and truly enjoys her meal. She says she eats very European: "For brunch, I might have a selection of fresh fruit, plain yogurt, cured beef, soy sausage, and various cheeses." She loves to cook grand meals for her friends, including fancy salad concoctions. Her favorite salads are avocado feta chicken with olive oil and lemon over butter lettuce and organic grilled vegetable salad.

Tracee's Organic Grilled Vegetable Salad

MAKES 2 GENEROUS SERVINGS

YOU WILL NEED
 A bundle of carrots
 A couple of zucchini
 Olive oil
 1 lemon slice
 1 head butter lettuce
 Balsamic goat cheese vinaigrette to taste

PREPARE
Season the carrots and zucchini with olive oil and lemon.
 Place in the broiler.
 When slightly crisp, place the carrots and zucchini on top of the lettuce.
 Dress with vinaigrette.
 Enjoy!

Liquid Yoga

The ancient art of healing by ingesting Chinese herbs is making a comeback and quickly traveling through the celebrity circuit. Elixir is Los Angeles's wildly popular herbal emporium, purveyor of herbs and elixirs, and a quiet, Zen-like oasis (plus, you are pretty much guaranteed to see a celebrity, such as Julia Roberts, Charlize Theron, Goldie Hawn, Heidi Klum, Penélope Cruz, Paula Abdul, or Jada Pinkett Smith, who have all been spotted there). Edgar Veytia, cofounder of Elixir, believes that "the whole notion of herbs is nutrition, beyond the basic food fuel group. Herbalism is a part of life. Eighty percent of the population depends on some sort of food or herbs for health care. Like food, herbalism is used out of necessity." People turn to herbs for a grab bag of reasons, from preventative medicine and antiaging to treatment of specific ailments or a lack of sex drive.

Many celebrities take home Elixir's top-notch herbs and tonics for stress reduction and mind-body balancing. "Celebrities like Elixir for a combination of the product and the atmosphere. Their appearance, vitality, and youthfulness are often the basis for their careers. We do get a lot of celebrities," admits Edgar. "Anybody who is anybody has been through here. But celebrities aren't the crux of our business. Stress affects everyone. It can have an all-around debilitating effect, and we are here to help fix that. No matter who you are." Basically, Elixir serves serenity in a cup through their tonics, herbal programs, and elixirs (my favorite is called Liquid Yoga).

Elixir is also known for its tea. In fact, it is not uncommon to see a dozen or so Angelenos lazing around in Elixir's garden sanctuary sipping tea and reading a book or jamming to the latest Zen music playing in their headphones. "Making tea is a lifestyle," says Edgar. "Tea is an extraordinary experience. It is very different from coffee, which is essentially a legal drug that people take every day. Tea doesn't seem to have as much gravitational pull. It is more introspective." Though Edgar may not believe that tea has a lot of "pull," Elixir tonics have been popping up at countless spas around the world. Spa goers are now being offered

Elixir's Virtual Buddha or Liquid Yoga to calm their nerves and relax their bodies before they step into their treatment rooms. "It's all about balance," notes Edgar. "Chinese medicine looks at lifestyle, age, and food, and then tries to put you back in balance in order to combat stressful situations with more ease. In ancient China, it was a terrible shame if a doctor's patient got sick. Herbalism is about how to stay well, not how to heal when you are sick. A cup of tea or a few herbal pills can help you achieve a blissful state of balance."

RESOURCES

www.coachjames.com
www.surlatable.com
www.wholefoodsmarket.com
www.lacosta.com
www.easydoesit.us
www.chefAkasha.com
www.foodnetwork.com
www.elixir.net
Elixir's Tonics & Teas by Jeff Stein and Edgar Veytia
Cooking the Real Age Way by Michael F. Roizen, M.D.,
    and John La Puma, M.D.
Health Solutions Stress Relief DVD from Gaiam
www.spiritualityforkids.com
www.llcuisine.com

Chapter Eight

You've Gotta Have Art

*Every child is an artist. The problem is how
to remain an artist once he grows up.*
—PABLO PICASSO

*When you make art, it slows you down.
You use the other part of your brain,
allowing you to focus on something that
is small and tangible, a detail that is calming,
a task that is accessible and that you can control.*
—MARCY WELLAND

COOL, SMOOTH molding clay warming as you knead it through your fingers . . . Broken tile shards fashioned into a mosaic frame . . . An ocean surfacing as delicate watercolors flow across the paper . . . A necklace emerging from a pile of glass beads. These are just a few of the reasons that the creation of art continues to be a satisfying serenity inducer for countless people.

Ed and Linda Buttwinick's Safe Haven Art Studio

Ed and Linda Buttwinick have worked with thousands of children and adults for the past thirty-two years as the founders and owners of the Brentwood Art Center in Los Angeles. The studio is also a safe haven for many Oscar- and Emmy-winning actors who seek out new ways to learn and grow as individuals as well as to expand their craft. According to Ed, who is also a painter, the sheer tactile experience of mixing the clay and rubbing paint into a canvas allows them to simultaneously get out of themselves and journey back into themselves with a renewed level of awareness. At the center there is no right and wrong, and no deadlines. Students are encouraged to create without rules and to make art that pleases themselves—not family or friends, and certainly not the public or fans. The many A-list celebrity moms who bring their children to the center also know that they are safe from the flashing cameras of the paparazzi. In fact, one Oscar-nominated actress recently told Buttwinick, "I come here because it's my sanctuary."

We all need to feel balanced and complete, and Ed knows that art feeds our spirits, releasing the inner imaginative self. Some people are drawn to art because of an innate need to use their hands, as well as a desire to communicate in a way other than through their lips. Others just want to have fun,

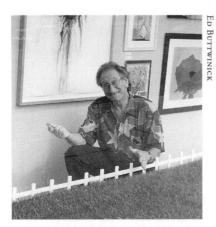

Ed Buttwinick at Brentwood Art Center.

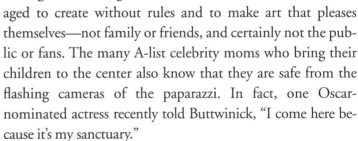
ED BUTTWINICK

see if they can do it, make something real or make an illusion, or test their hand-eye coordination. The reasons that people begin to paint, sculpt, or craft are as individual as the finished products.

Jane Seymour's Stress-Releasing Refuge

Painting is Jane Seymour's "refuge." She painted between takes while on *Dr. Quinn, Medicine Woman*. When she is restless at night or coping with turbulence on an airplane, drawing is her meditation. What started out as finger painting with her children has turned into a passion and a vocation for this actress who has more than fifty television shows and films to her credit.

Art on the Go

Marcy Welland, who along with her husband, Al, owns Art On The Go, a company that "brings art projects to you," has found that the more hectic the world has become, the more people want to get back to less complicated times, and nothing is as basic as feeling paint squish through your fingers. Unfortunately, many of us stopped making art after childhood. Yet there is a longing to return to the innocence of paper, pencils, and paint. According to Marcy, "When you make art, it slows you down. You use the other part of your brain, allowing you to focus on something that is small and tangible, a detail that is calming, a task that is accessible and that you can control." Completing an art project, either for yourself or as a

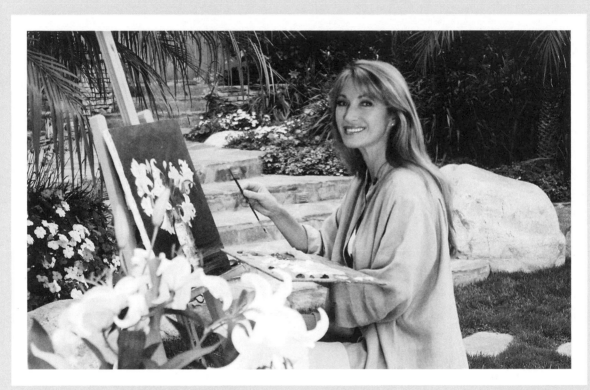

Jane Seymour at her easel.

gift, gives you a tremendous sense of accomplishment. Although Jane says, "I paint for myself," she also loves giving her creations as gifts. While working on *Dr. Quinn,* the actress painted on T-shirts, often giving them to the crew as presents.

Initially self-taught, Jane felt more confident as she began to learn painting skills. She looked at great art books, copied her favorite artists, and learned techniques from the masters. She recommends starting with watercolor painting. Use the best watercolor blocks, such as Winsor & Newton, buy sable brushes and four-hundred-pound pressed paper with torn edges. Another good way to begin, according to Jane, is with pastels. "They are very forgiving; you can mush them around with your fingers."

According to Marcy, celebrities, including actors, producers, and directors, are turning to art as a way to relieve stress because it allows them to let go, be themselves, and not play a role. The day-to-day details disappear and concentration is on the tactile experience. When Marcy and Al had a storefront operation called Create Your Own, their celebrity clientele, including Catherine Hicks and Vanna White, would find themselves lost in the making of art, totally free from the demands of a ticking clock.

Lauren Holly's Artistic Addiction

What started as a hobby between takes on the sets of films including *What Women Want, Any Given Sunday,* and *Dumb & Dumber* has turned into an addiction for the actress Lauren Holly. Not to worry, it is a healthy addiction, a stress-relieving addiction in fact, that preserves wonderful memories in a book. Now Lauren has a suitcase filled with scrapbooking supplies that she takes with her when she travels. Scrapbooking is not a project that ends; it continuously records your life as you live it. Says Lauren, "Scrapbooking, for me, started because my nanny was into it. She was a great photographer, and she would shoot images while we were on location for a film, and then we would drink wine and scrapbook them."

For Lauren, scrapbooking has also become a social event. "It is a time when you can get together with other women. Plus, when I am scrapbooking things for my children, I like that I am being a great mom!" Lauren goes on, "Now, scrapbooking has turned into such an obsession that we have a room in my house dedicated to it!" She also turns some of her mini scrapbook pages into decoupage. She says, "Though I make photo albums mainly, I have made collages and family picture frames. I give them as gifts and little mementos."

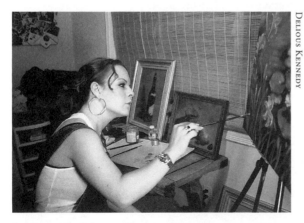

Jenna von Oy in her studio.

Delious Kennedy

Jenna von Oy's Room Devoted to Crafts

Jenna von Oy, who stars on *The Parkers,* also paints. For years, she says, she was "aching to have a room devoted to crafts" after her boyfriend gave her an easel and paints for Valentine's Day with a note: "I didn't want to stifle your creativity." Jenna has enrolled in painting classes at O'Neill's Fine Art Studio in Malibu and spends hours engrossed in her personal sacred space. Although she gets inspiration from many sources, including the memorabilia, journals, paintings, and travel mementos that are in her studio, she likes the idea of taking a class to improve her skill.

Nicole Ritchie's Artistic Antics

Nicole Ritchie, famous for her party-girl antics and *Simple Life* mischief, lives a simpler life than you might imagine. Proficient in three instruments—the piano, violin, and cello—Nicole has undoubtedly inherited some of her father's musical genius. "I play all the time," she reveals with a calm smile on her face. "My dad taught me. But I can't read music, my dad can't either, so I play by ear. When my dad was writing music we would just sit down and play for hours and hours. We still do it now." Musicians are known to get lost in their music. Stress seeps through the notes allowing for a rush of rapture.

Ballet is another of Nicole's solace-providing passions. "I started ballet at three years old. My dad wrote 'Ballerina Girl' for me," she says with a smile. "I used to dance all the time. But I really don't do it much anymore." For the time being, Nicole has swapped her toe shoes for a pen as she writes her album. "I have always been a writer. Writing music is not something that you start doing or learn, it is something that you do. I write the instrumental since I am not a lyricist."

As Nicole walks down the street in stiletto heels, the entrance to the chicest club to hit the scene just steps away, she knows that while baby blue and pink dyed hair may extend from her head, creativity oozes from her being.

Asha Blake's Artist Break from Journalism

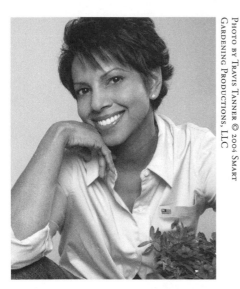

Photo by Travis Tanner © 2004 Smart Gardening Productions, LLC

Asha Blake

Asha Blake, a television journalist who has hosted NBC's *Later Today,* the nationally syndicated show *Life Moments,* and ABC's *World News Now,* spends her "me-time" hand-coloring black-and-white photographs she has taken. Before her daughter was born, Asha's time for herself included all kinds of exercise, from Rollerblading to lifting weights and dancing. A definite shift in activities occurred after Sasha's birth, and while Asha prefers to alleviate the pressures of the day with some exercise, she also enjoys cooking, gardening, photography, and hand-tinting photographs. She learned to hand-tint from Sally Gray, a neighbor from her husband Mark's hometown in Minnesota.

For all of her career Asha has "interviewed people to hear their inner thoughts, and studied their faces." She loves photography because it allows her to read who a person is at a given moment in time. Asha started earnestly making photos five years ago while taking pictures of her daughter. Soon after she discovered color tinting and has since spent as much time as she can in her guest bedroom—studio, alone, after 11:00 P.M. When her family has gone to sleep, Asha enjoys "not talking" for once, and she allows her mind to wander, welcoming the rush of thoughts. Working into the night, she finds joy in anticipating how happy the people in her photographs will be when they see how lovingly she has tinted their images. Asha works on a big artist drawing table. She is inspired by two hand-tinted photographs, both of which were

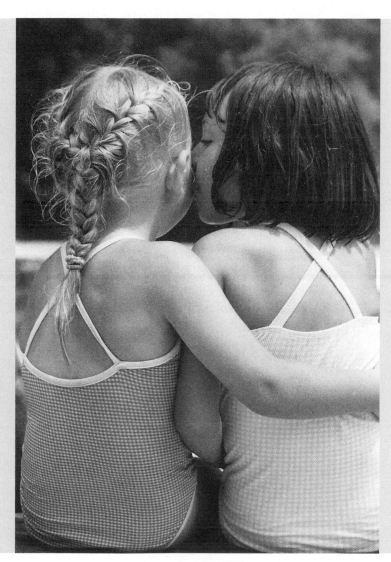

Original hand-tinted photograph by Asha Blake.

done by her "guru" Sally. During those late-night sessions, she lights a scented candle and sometimes watches *Inside the Actors Studio.* But more often, she just basks in the silence, knowing that the telephone isn't going to ring, at least until the sun comes up.

Each of Asha's photographs represents a special moment in time; however, the journey of the first photo she hand-tinted is especially meaningful. While living in New York and working at NBC, Asha tinted a portrait of her friend's daughter Amanda. Amanda's mom, Daniela, proudly displayed the photo on her desk in her office, located across from the World Trade Center. The photo was so striking that fellow employees often commented on it. When Daniela's building was severely damaged on September 11, 2001, she thought that the eight-by-ten photo was lost forever. But months later, after a journey that touched the lives of many recovering from the tragedy, the photo arrived in an envelope, virtually unscathed. Apparently after the dusty photo was found, everyone who saw it knew its owner . . . Daniela.

Asha has read numerous books on photography and hand tinting, studied countless photos, and taken many classes. The Web site www.handcolor.com lists classes, articles, and sources. Find a class in your area and choose subject matter that interests you. For Asha, the subject matter is always people, especially children, because she loves to capture "that special moment in a child's day."

Janet Gunn's Homemade Jewels

The actress Janet Gunn discovered jewelry making when she was starring in CBS's *Dark Justice* in 1992. Shooting mostly at night, Janet was always drained of energy and desperate to discover something to help her make it through the long nights. She went to a bead store, purchased some stones, and began a hobby that has turned into Janet Gunn Designs, with a clientele that includes Meredith Brooks, Carrie-Anne Moss, and Kathleen Quinlan.

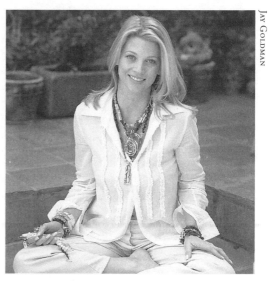

Janet Gunn with her jewelry.

Before jewelry making became a business, however, it was a stress-reducing salvation for Janet as she went from *Dark Justice* to *Silk Stalkings* to *CSI* to feature films, including a three-month location shoot on *The Quest* with Jean-Claude Van Damme in Thailand. As soon as she started beading, time flew by. She says, "I had no thoughts, it was like meditation for me." The instant gratification of completing a necklace, coupled with the joy of giving the jewelry as gifts, started the actress on a new career path. After September 11, she realized that she wasn't fulfilled. Jewelry designing had filled a void, giving her satisfaction as well as serenity. Her priorities had changed, and with a lot of encouragement from her friends, she turned the hobby into a career. Janet's friend Meredith Brooks wears the jewelry on tour because, she boasts, "it is unique and cool. . . . I know that I have something nobody else does." Calling it the "sexy, cool Janet style,"

Gems from Janet on Jewelry Designing

If it is something you want to do, don't find reasons not to do it.

Go to a craft store, bead store, or button store; pick out your favorite colors.

Have an open mind.

Remember it's your creation. No one is telling you what to do.

Even if you think you are not creative, when you sit down, remember that what you are making is an expression of something you haven't tapped into before.

Keep the motivation.

If it is possible, find a place in your home that is a "sacred work space," a place all your own.

Meredith feels that the collection helps her define her image while offering a selection of perfect gifts for her hard-to-please celebrity friends.

Janet is inspired by color and works with all natural products, including semiprecious stones, silver, and gold. Each piece is a balance between strength (represented by the metals), femininity, and vulnerability (epitomized by the stones). Her studio, a tiny space in her garage, is her refuge. Stimulated by music, the scent of cut roses from her garden, orange blossoms floating in water, and candles, Janet is able to distance herself from the Hollywood rat race and create stunning designs that are sexy and cool, at least by Meredith Brooks's standards!

Grown-up Art Parties

Social interaction and a sense of community can also serve as rewards of the practice of creating art. Many of Marcy Welland's clients are asking her to create art experiences for them, with friends, in the privacy of their own homes. Group quilting lessons, jewelry-making sessions, and

Grown-Up Craft Parties, Courtesy of Art On The Go

Have a preplanning session: Gather friends, have snacks, and jot down what you would like to accomplish each month.

Create a workable schedule. Will you gather once a month? Every other month? Each participant chooses a date to host. The host organizes the evening, provides the location, snacks, and supplies. Specify ground rules: No cell phones? No children?

On the designated evening, the art supplies should be available on a large table, with clean-up supplies nearby.

Here are some easy projects:

Decoupage boxes. Supplies include balsa wood or cardboard boxes, papers, photos, magazines that can be torn, and glue.

Jewelry. Supplies include beads, stretchy elastic, and clasps.

Decorative candles. Supplies include candles, dried flowers, glue, and tweezers.

Potpourri sachet. Supplies include dried rosemary or other aromatic herbs or flowers, mesh bags, ribbon, and tulle.

"grown-up craft parties" are replacing traditional cocktail parties and wedding showers. During these grown-up get-togethers, cell phones and pagers are turned off and conversation takes center stage. The focus becomes whether to use the green paper or the blue paper instead of the kids' problems, the freeway commute, or office issues. Conversations often take a turn, as memories surface and guests begin to connect, letting go of the stresses of the day.

Decoupage, the art of applying photos and paper to papier-mâché, wood, walls, and other surfaces is, according to Marcy, a safe project for a beginner group. It is easy, virtually mistake-free, and the supplies are readily available. Local arts and craft stores such as Michael's and Ben Franklin, as well as various bookstores, sell art books with simple decoupage instructions.

Ed believes that the need to create, whether it is art or music, is spiritually and emotionally essential. Maybe for some the smell of turpentine or the feel of clay between the fingers doesn't conjure up such feeling. However, for those to whom it is enticing, he has some recommendations:

- Start from a place of interest. It's okay to dabble. If you are interested in clay, play in the dirt. If you are drawn to color, tear pieces of colored paper and arrange them in a pattern that pleases you.
- Choose what pleases you and what you have fun with. Select what feels right. You need the right key to open up the door to art.
- Go to an art or craft store and buy some supplies.
- Seek help from a mentor, a class, or maybe a book.
- Look at art. Go to galleries and museums.

- Copy other artists, but go beyond them; it is too narrow a road just to copy.
- Have fun.
- Remember that you are never too old. Ed's mother-in-law, at age eighty, has discovered watercolor painting and now buys fruit not based on taste but according to their color.
- You are only required to please yourself.

When Ed wants to escape from the constant stimulation of the Brentwood Art Center, he finds sanctuary in his studio next to the Santa Monica Airport. There, he enters a world that, he says, "is my own, filled with my life history." In complete silence, except for the occasional drone of an airplane as it lands next to his window, he creates, surrounded by the items that stimulate him—boxes of broken toys and pieces of random equipment, old pens, masks, vintage televisions, and loads of other stuff that many would consider junk. Each item is categorized and placed in a plastic box so the artist can call on them when needed. Inspired by his heritage, Ed creates assemblages and artworks from this random assortment of objects.

The ability of art to transport us from our everyday existence, the minutiae that exhaust us, the bosses who constantly look over our shoulders, or the toddlers tugging at our pant legs, is the key to its capacity to save our sanity. Art makes us whole.

RESOURCES

Two of Ed Buttwinick's favorite books are *The Natural Way to Draw* by Kim
 Nicolaides and *Drawing Lessons from the Great Masters* by Robert
 Beverly Hale
Remarkably Changes by Jane Seymour
www.brentwoodart.com
www.handcolor.com

Chapter Nine

Nurturing Nature

*Gardening is an active participation in
the deeper mysteries of the universe.*
—THOMAS BERRY

THERE IS SOMETHING so healing that happens when you cultivate your very own garden. Nurturing a life, be it in a hundred-acre field or a simple four-inch pot, can create an incredible sense of responsibility and accomplishment. So plant a garden, or a single stem of your favorite flower or herb. Many people get excited to go outside and water, to see the changes and the growth, and finally to harvest a few basil leaves to add to a dinner, a mint leaf to punctuate a dessert, or the sweetest-smelling rose to enrich the bedroom.

My (Sharon) Mecca is my garden. More than receiving a soothing massage or taking an inspiring yoga class, sitting among my flowers and succulents soothes my soul. It's somewhat of a miracle that I embrace gardening, since my early memories of things growing included my father insisting that I mow the lawn and weed the garden every Saturday, without regard to my hay fever. Now, nothing is more relaxing for me than planting a new lobelia or even skimming the muck from my tiny pond. Whenever I travel to New York City, my only required indulgence is to stay at a hotel that faces one of the world's greatest gardens—Central Park.

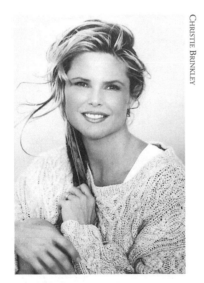

Christie Brinkley

Christie Brinkley's Spirit Replenished

Martha Stewart isn't the only one who makes a living out of gardening; the supermodel Christie Brinkley does too, though instead of making a *financial* living, Christie makes a life. After years of living in the fast lane as a highly paid, in-demand model, Christie has found pleasure in her garden. She says that "when I focus on any one of my million hobbies, any stress and tension I may have been feeling simply vanishes. But it is gardening above all else that completely replenishes my spirit. Sometimes, I enter my garden in a frazzled state, but the second I pick up a rake, shovel, or clippers and set to my chores, I fall into a Zen-like state of peacefulness and contentment. I am serenaded by the birds and caressed by the sun and breeze. Any doubt in my heart is reassured by the new growth and buds. Each blossom is a celebration. I have taught my children how to garden and nurture, and now they share the same joy and appreciation. When we enter our garden at dawn and are still gardening under the moonlight, we look at one another and say, 'What a perfect day!' "

Amber Valletta's Weekend Weeding

Perhaps it's the constant striving for perfection inherent in the world of supermodeling that makes gardening such a relief. The übermodel Amber Valletta enjoys nothing better than a "weeding weekend" with her fiancé. She says, "We pull weeds and cut flowers on the weekends when I am home. It is wonderful to see things grow. We have so much fruit that we could open a small grocery store. But instead, we eat it."

Gardens engage all of our senses. From the delicate scent of a rose that reminds you of your grandmother's perfume to a tiny sage plant that evokes memories of Thanksgiving family gatherings, plants trigger memories. If you listen carefully, gardens also serve as an auditory delight—the ever-so-subtle flapping of butterfly wings, the rustling leaves in a gentle breeze, and the buzzing of a bee as it alights on your lavender plant. The many treats for your senses all contribute to the serenity-boosting powers of gardening.

Art Luna's Garden Salon

Art Luna, whose West Hollywood hair salon is frequented by a myriad of stars, including Priscilla Presley, Anjelica Huston, and Kelly Lynch, has been so seduced by the joys of gardening that he has become a hyphenate—a gardener-hairdresser. The metamorphosis from high-powered hair wizard to garden designer took place when Art's beauty business was bustling. Slowly, his salon and garden became one, and Art found that his clients loved to sit among the flowering pots on his patio, listening to the melodic fountains as they waited for their color to set. The transformation makes perfect sense to Art: "Gardens are all about color, shape, texture, and proportion—the segue from hairstylist to gardener required the same appreciation." Clients began to ask questions about the foliage, and suddenly the conversation was not about their hair but rather about his plants!

Gradually, Art even began to assist his clients with their gardens, including his friend the actress and *The West Wing* star Stockard Channing, who admired the blooms at his salon. Sharing a love for fluid lines, hot colors, and adventurous breeds, the two began to scout nurseries to fill his growing plot as well as her cottage garden. Art believes that the relationship worked because they were both willing to experiment, knowing that a garden isn't a museum but rather a living, breathing thing, with a soul. He explains, "We look at the garden very much the way a painter perceives his or her canvas. We learn from each other about texture and color. I know she likes unusual architectural shapes, like me. She knows what colors feel right and loves wonderful hot color combinations, as I do. We aren't afraid

Art Luna's Recipe for Starting a Garden

First, find your area, be it a yard, patio, house, or balcony.

Decide whether you want to live in the space or simply look at it.

Visit lots of gardens, not just garden supply stores. See how gardeners work with various colors.

Find the plants you like. Determine if they are right for your personal space.

Do research. Buy books. Personal favorites include *Garden Design* by David Hicks and *The Education of a Gardener* by Russell Page, which helped me understand tradition and structure.

Remember that a garden is living, growing, and evolving. Don't be afraid of it.

to experiment. So together, we have created a cottage garden that is perfectly suited to Stockard."

Gardens change . . . constantly. Sometimes a plant works, and sometimes it doesn't. Art relishes the relinquishing of control that his garden offers. For him, "it's almost scary how fast time goes by in the garden." Art doesn't believe that it is necessary to be trained in garden design, in fact, self-taught gardeners who have a background in painting and design have created most of the gardens that he loves.

Katherine Whiteside, the "Garden Goddess"

Even goddesses love to garden. Katherine Whiteside, the "Garden Goddess" for *House Beautiful,* practices what she preaches. An authority on gardens whose work includes serving as the national garden adviser and spokesperson for Smith and Hawken, Katherine loves nothing better than to spend time in her own garden. She says that when she is "feeling aggravated and nervous and dwelling on myself," she goes to her garden, where "I can get out of myself. I go outside to forget about me. Just doing the physical labor, like picking a flower, is meditative." Pleasing yourself is an essential part of creating a pleasant garden, as well as starting small, according to Katherine. One way that you can "start small" is a container garden—a collection of your favorite pots (either indoors or outside) arranged in a pleasant pattern. "After all, if the plant dies, at least you still have the pot," muses Katherine. Although she advocates the use of interesting containers, she acknowledges that keeping it simple, using a limited color palette or concentrating on a specific material, such as clay, wood, or metal, can be soothing. In her very helpful book, *Forcing, etc.,* Katherine demonstrates how easy it is to begin a garden.

Katherine's Top Ten Gardening Tips

1. Before you begin each season, mark ideas you like in gardening books. A nice array of sticky notes always marks a good garden.

2. The real key to garden success is *start small*. It's fun to realize that next season you can take on more. It is discouraging to realize that, from the very beginning, you are overwhelmed.

3. Go organic. It is better for you, your kids, and your pets. And it is actually easier and far less expensive. Planting natural pesticides such as rosemary, basil, and fern leaf marigolds next to bug magnets is also helpful.

4. Grow a small vegetable garden. Even two tomato plants and a basil bush will make a huge difference in your garden enjoyment.

5. Make a tiny cutting garden. Plant easy annuals like zinnias, sunflowers, and bachelor's buttons. You'll always have flowers for the house and to give away.

6. Don't make your kids work in your garden. Remember Tom Sawyer's fence painting techniques and you'll have children who will always enjoy puttering in the garden.

7. Don't worry about having a lawn like a golf course. It looks fake and takes too many chemicals. Enjoy an imperfect lawn, where your kids and pets can frolic.

8. Eat outside whenever possible. Have one sunny spot for morning coffee and another larger table for family meals and entertaining.

9. Buy comfortable garden chairs. After a day of gardening, you should always take time to sit down and admire your handiwork.

10. Think of your garden as a work of art in progress. Don't fret over tiny imperfections, but enjoy all the progress you have made. A garden is a great place to think hopeful thoughts.

Katherine's Soothing Sage Sachet

Gather fresh sage from your pots or garden.

Either dry in the sun or use fresh.
Pack the leaves in a small muslin bag. These are often found near the tea
section at your local market.
Add fresh orange peel.
Seal and place in the tub for a calming bath.

Joie Cosentino's Healing Gardens

Joie Cosentino comes from a long line of gardeners. Her family's Cosentino Nursery has been a fixture in Malibu for more than thirty years. Legions of celebrities have been sighted at the nursery, which has grown to multiple locations. From Liberace, who surrounded himself with beautiful flowers and orchids, to Keely Shaye Smith, who loves vegetables and herbs (always organic), Cosentino's has been an institution for celebrities who find solace in their gardens. Barbra Streisand, with her exquisite taste and extensive knowledge about gardens, personally shops for the plants, flowering pinks and whites, which make up her garden. And Ed Harris often shows up in his truck, personally selecting and schlepping the plants that encompass his and his wife Amy Madigan's garden.

"Gardening repairs the soul," according to Joie. "When you are in the

Joie's Recipe for Starting a Garden

Don't challenge yourself too much. Start with a hearty plant, perhaps one that will reward you with a bloom. The kalanchoe, a blooming plant that can take sun and shade, is a favorite. It won't make you feel discouraged.

After you have success with the first plant, try another—maybe one that is more complicated.

The best gardeners are willing to put in the time.

Use good judgment. You must observe your plants. Don't water according to a timetable. If the plant is drooping, it needs to be watered, even if it's off schedule.

garden, the focus is on the plant, which you need to care for. Only your care guarantees its survival. Plants closely resemble children; everything they get, they get from their parents. When a plant blooms, we, like parents, feel rewarded."

Mark Giebel's Garden

Mark Giebel, whose family has owned Mordigan's nursery, a thirty-seven-year-old staple for celebrities from James Stewart and Vincent Price to Millie Perkins and Patricia Heaton, feels that the sheer act of pausing for a moment to take in all the colors at a nursery is enough for some people.

The actress Moon Unit Zappa, in a 2001 *New York Times* article

Mark's Recipe for Starting a Garden

Start small.

Have a plan.

Purchase color packs, 6 to 12 colorful flowering stems.

Radishes give the beginning gardener instant gratification.

Bulbs are great because you can literally watch them grow, particularly if they are planted in glass containers.

Chives in a Pot

Standard potting mixture

Terra-cotta pot

Chive seeds

Plenty of sunshine

The chives will begin to germinate in 6 to 8 days, guaranteeing instant satisfaction.

entitled "One Street at a Time: Positively Third Street," waxed enthusiastic about Mordigan's, a full-service nursery nestled in busy, urban West Hollywood. The actress offered this interesting and thought-provoking tidbit: "Seriously, what better way to spend lazing around an overcast weekend in the city than at a nursery? It is next to impossible to be in a bad mood around plants."

A Personal Herb Garden

10-inch terra-cotta pot
Planter's soil
1 basil plant for cooking
1 peppermint plant for cooking, using in baths, and simply for a relaxing whiff
1 herb of your choice

Water every other day.
Visit every day.
Enjoy the herbs by using them in cooking and bathing.
Once the herbs are flourishing, you can either dry or freeze them and enjoy the fruits of your labor for months to come.

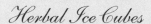

Herbal Ice Cubes

Add fresh-snipped herbs, such as basil, tarragon, or thyme, to a plastic ice cube tray.
Gently pour spring or filtered water over the herbs.
Freeze and enjoy.

This is the perfect way to preserve your fresh herbs. When you want to use the herbs, either melt them or pop the cubes into cold water for a refreshing herbal drink.

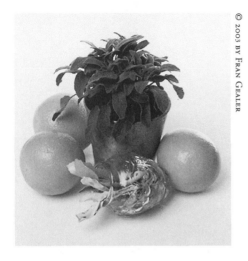

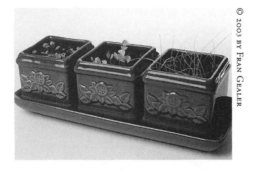

Mark feels that herb gardens are perfect projects for beginners. Not only are they satisfying but they can also enhance your kitchen and bathroom. Be creative. Are you interested in butterflies, Italian cooking, biblical references, or the color purple? Herb gardens can be tailor-made to fit any theme. They can be planted in terra-cotta pots, wooden planters, large tin cans, or cast-off pottery. One of the easiest herbs to grow is chives.

A Sanctuary Garden

A sanctuary garden is a meditative space that grows and changes with the seasons and is the perfect refuge for relaxation and reflection. From a collection of pots nestled on the patio and filled with fragrant herbs and colorful annuals to a sculpted garden such as the one created by my friend Gail that occupies an acre in Hollywood, a sanctuary garden provides peace and calm. Wind chimes, tiny sculptures, and flags are the perfect addition to any sanctuary garden. Gail's more elaborate design includes an homage to the sculptor Beatrice Wood with platforms embedded with lusterware, a performance area (home to impromptu jazz concerts during the summer months), and artistic odes to a range of philosophers and artists.

Starting a Sanctuary Garden

First, visualize the space.

Sit in a comfortable chair where you plan to place your garden.

Write down your thoughts. What do you hope to experience in this space?

Conceptualize the entrance, colors, plants, sculpture, and accessories.

Do you want to sit in the garden, walk through it, or simply stand?

What is your budget?

Once this preplanning has been completed, it is time to turn the hoe!

RESOURCES

Garden Design by David Hicks

The Education of a Gardener by Russell Page

www.smithandhawken.com

Forcing, etc. by Katherine Whiteside

The Sanctuary Garden by Christopher Forrest McDowell and Tricia Clark-McDowell

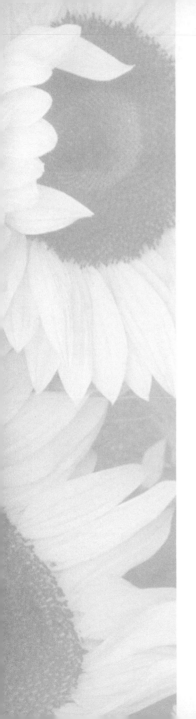

Chapter Ten

Knit One, Purl Too

I crochet in the hairdresser's chair and
even behind the puzzle board.
I can get out of myself when I crochet.
— VANNA WHITE

Edith Eig Arouses Impassioned Knitting

"I can't stop . . . I don't have the time to stop . . . My car stops automatically at your shop . . . I have to stop in. I have the intention to come in for only a few minutes, and I end up spending the afternoon!" What has this Emmy nominated star so impassioned? Knitting is her fix, and Edith Eig, the proprietor of La Knitterie Parisienne in Studio City, California, is this comedienne's guru.

Walking into Edith's store is a sensory experience; the walls are loaded with skeins of yarn in every imaginable colorand texture. The sound of chatter from the women sitting around a big oval table is comforting: "I dropped my stitch." "My scarf is too long." "What needle should I use for this stitch?" "Does my jerk of a boyfriend deserve this hat?" This is a typical day at the shop, with women of all ages gathered for a dose of knitting therapy.

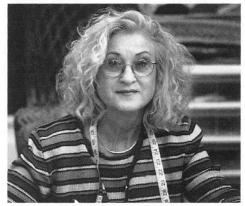

On any given day the group will include actresses such as Sarah Michelle Gellar, Mary Kate and Ashley Olsen, Jennifer Connelly, Kristin Davis, Daryl Hannah, and Caroline Rhea, their mothers, agents, producers, and everyone else, all showing off their latest knitting creations. They also seek camaraderie from the group and advice from the master. On this particular afternoon, Alex, an

Edith Eig of La Knitterie Parisienne.

actress pregnant with her first child, says of knitting, "It's something I can do on the set." Chimes in another, "It beats smoking." Edith's motto is "As you knit, so shall you rip," acknowledging that mistakes are made and patience is required.

Justine Bateman Designs

Justine Bateman, best known for her years on *Family Ties,* was so taken by knitting and her experience with Edith that she launched Justine Bateman Designs, a collection of hand-knitted sweaters and accessories. According to Eig, the actress discovered that the craft sparked all sorts of ideas, and she found in Edith a mentor and friend. "Edith is incredibly helpful and giving of her knitting skills and experience," states the actress. "I wouldn't know much about knitting without her."

Edith feels that it is the "hurry up and wait" nature of television and motion picture production that draws so many celebrities to knitting. "They have lots of idle time on their hands between takes on the set and while they are in the makeup chair." Knitting doesn't require full time, and it certainly helps to pass the hours. And, says Edith, it's a great mother-daughter activity. *Buffy the Vampire Slayer*'s Sarah Michelle Gellar, who became proficient after one fifteen-minute session, often comes to the store with her mother. The actress is so devoted to knitting that her agent, not knowing what else to give her on her twenty-sixth birthday, came up with a gift certificate to La Knitterie Parisienne.

Knitting as Therapy

The actress Daryl Hannah always wanted to knit but never thought she could until she met Edith. "Her patience and kindness have opened up a whole new world for me," states Daryl, who loves the meditative and repetitive quality of knitting. Caroline Rhea, who claims that Edith "can take you from pot holder to cable-knit sweater in no time," calls her the "Deepak Chopra of knitting." Another actress claims that, before going into an audition, she stops to knit, stating, "It gives me karma." According to Edith, the therapeutic values of knitting are endless. And although it might not cure the common cold (unless the cold is related to stress), knitting offers many serenity-inducing qualities:

- Concentrates your mind on the knitting, not on your problems
- Focuses your energy on creativity

- Is relaxing, indulgent, and therapeutic
- Provides a meditative and peaceful rhythm
- Serves as a creative outlet
- Stimulates and exercises the mind
- Offers a sense of accomplishment—you can wear your artwork
- Teaches discipline and patience
- Provides continuity

Edith's Recipe to Begin Knitting

Find a good knitting store. Most communities have one. The store's owner should be happy to provide instruction.

Start with something simple but not boring. Check out local department stores and boutiques. Study the knitted pieces and ask questions. A scarf is a good first project. Think about making a simple gift for a friend (having a recipient in mind is often good motivation).

Use smooth, high-quality yarn. Choose yarn that excites you and appeals to your sense of touch.

Smooth needles, such as bamboo, are easier for the beginner because they don't slip.

Find a good book.

Find or start a knitting group.

Tune in to my show, *Knit One, Purl Two: A Knitting Workshop with Edith Eig,* on DIY—Do It Yourself Network.

Although it's difficult to learn to knit by reading a book, a few simple knitting terms are essential:

- *Knitting:* Forming rows of interconnecting loops in which the ends of the loops face away from you as you work. Your needle is inserted from front to back.
- *Purling:* Forming rows of interconnecting loops in which the ends of the loops face toward you as you work. The needle is inserted from back to front. Many devotees also follow the chant, "In, over, through, and off."

If, like Debra Messing, you find that the yearning to use yarn overtakes you, Edith has a simple scarf recipe that is certain to please. In fact, Jennie Garth, Daryl Hannah, Julianne Margulies, Sarah Michelle Gellar, and Ashley Olsen are all working on scarves. With their long, slim length and

Edith's Recipe for a Scarf

MATERIALS NEEDED

3 balls of Kross yarn

Size 11 needles

Scarf will measure 8 inches across.

Sand stitch (ideal for this scarf because it is reversible)

Row 1: Knit across.

Row 2: Knit 1, purl 1 across.

Repeat these two rows until you reach your desired length.

chunky stitch, scarves are at the height of fashion. The basic garter stitch makes knitting a scarf easy, and Edith's celebrity clients individualize their fashions by combining unusual colors with metallic yarn for a texture that is bright, soft, and in many cases, very hairy. Creating a scarf is a wonderful mother-daughter activity because the repetitive stitches don't require much concentration. Dakota Fanning and her mother, as well as Sarah Michelle Gellar and her mom, spend many an hour at the shop engaged in conversation as they gauge their stitches.

For the slightly more advanced student, such as the actress Laura Leighton, Edith likes a tote bag.

Edith's Recipe for a Tote Bag

MATERIALS NEEDED
  3 skeins Tahki Baby Print
  Size 17 needles
  Markers
  Stockinette stitch
  Gauge: 2 stitches = 1 inch

Make two pieces, front and back.
  Cast on 19 stitches.
  Beginning with a purl row, work in stockinette for 5 rows.
  Cable cast on 4 stitches, knit across.
  Cast on 4 stitches and purl across.

Next row, knit 4, place a marker, slip 1 purlwise, place a marker, knit to the last 5 stitches, place a marker, slip 1 purlwise, knit 4, purl back.

Repeat these 2 rows 11 times, or 22 rows.

Next row, remove a marker, knit 6 more rows in stockinette.

Bind off loosely.

HANDLE

Cast on 9 stitches.

Purl 1 row.

Next row, knit 2, place a marker, slip 1, place a marker, knit 3, place a marker, slip 1, place a marker, knit 2.

Purl 1 row.

Repeat these 2 rows 17 times, or 34 rows.

Bind off loosely.

FINISHING

Sew all sides together and sew handle into place. Join seams along row ends and cast on edges. Attach handle inside upper edges (approximately 2.5 inches from side seams).

OPTIONAL FINISHING

Lining and inside zipper pocket. For the lining, you have your choice of fabric, measured to the size of the finished bag. Reverse bag and sew lining into place. Use a zipper to create a pocket sewn into the lining.

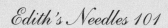

Edith's Needles 101

To fully understand how to knit, one must have a working knowledge of needles and stitches—the basics, according to Edith, of the craft. Quite simply, needles fall into two categories: wood and metal. Choosing a needle is strictly a matter of preference, although metal needles tend to be slightly slicker than their wooden counterparts, and Edith doesn't recommend them for beginners. In the world of needles, size matters; needle size dictates the type of stitch and thus the type of product that is created.

Wooden Needles: Bamboo, rosewood, ebony

Turbo or Metal Needles: Nickel plated, can be very slick

Edith's Yarn 101

Five categories of yarn are available.

FINGERING YARN

7 stitches per inch

Needs size 2–3 needle

Comes in synthetic and natural (wool, silk)

SPORT OR DOUBLE KNITTING (DK) YARN

6 stitches per inch

Needs size 5–6 needle

Comes in synthetic and natural

WORSTED OR ARAN
   4½-5 stitches per inch
   Needs size 7-8 needle
   Comes in synthetic and natural

CHUNKY
   3-3½ stitches per inch
   Needs size 10½-11 needle
   Comes in synthetic and natural

SUPER CHUNKY
   1–2½ stitches per inch
   Needs size 13–plus needle
   Comes in synthetic and natural

Super Chunky yarn is the rage now with actresses because it is great for ponchos and superfuzzy scarves.

Vanna White Finds Time to Crochet Behind the Wheel

Vanna White has legions of fans from *Wheel of Fortune.* However, before she was a mega-television star, there was crocheting. Her grandmother crocheted, and at the age of five Vanna started chain stitching, using the required tools of crocheting—yarn and a crochet hook. Her love of crocheting followed her to the set of *Wheel of Fortune,* where Vanna recalls,

"I crochet in the hairdresser's chair and even behind the puzzle board." While she was navigating through a rocky patch in her life, crocheting helped to preserve Vanna's serenity because, she says, "It's therapeutic. I can get out of myself when I crochet. I'm in another world. I don't have to think, and I don't have to count like with knitting."

Vanna also loves to give crocheted gifts to friends. "What do you give to someone who has everything?" In the case of Merv Griffin, ten years ago, it was a handmade afghan. Baby gifts, from afghans and blankets to booties and frames, are also favorites of the actress. Vanna has taken her love for crocheting one step further with the publication of four books for

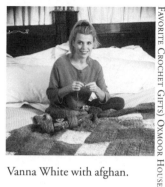

Vanna White with afghan.

A Favorite Frame from Vanna
(excerpted from Vanna's Favorite Crochet Gifts)

YOU WILL NEED

A picture frame

Sport-weight yarn, approximately
1¾ ounces (195 yards), variegated

Size G crochet hook

2 yards each ³⁄₁₆-inch-wide picot-edged
ribbons in favorite pastel colors

Various baby trinkets

Craft glue

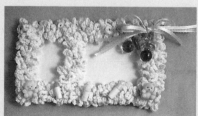

Vanna White's favorite frame.

Oxmoor House. A favorite fairly simple recipe for a baby frame is included in *Vanna's Favorite Crochet Gifts*. Although this isn't a traditional crocheted item, it is so easy that even a novice should be able to succeed.

Liza Huber's Needlepoint Passion

Like Vanna, Liza Huber, one of the stars of the daytime drama *Passions*, has discovered the benefits of stitching her stress away. She has turned to needlepoint to stop what her fiancé calls "the hamster wheel in her head." She does it on planes and before bed and also loves to give needlepoint pieces as gifts. One of her favorites is "a needlepoint of a 1920s movie star lying on the floor writing love letters and smoking a cigarette out of one of those long plastic holders."

RESOURCES

The Knitters Companion by Vicki Square

Hip to Knit by Judith L. Swartz

Knitting Lessons: Tales from the Knotting Path by Lela Nargi

Zen and the Art of Knitting by Bernadette Murphy

The Complete Idiot's Guide to Knitting and Crocheting by Gail Diven and Cindy Kitchel

Vanna's Favorite Crochet Gifts by Vanna White

Vanna's Afghans A to Z by Vanna White

Vanna's Afghans All Through the House by Vanna White

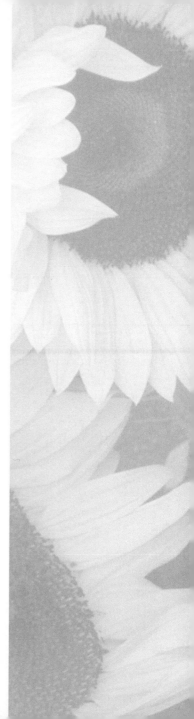

Chapter Eleven

Sacred Spaces and Feng Shui

> *There is no need to go to India or*
> *anywhere to find peace. You will find that*
> *deep place of silence right in your room,*
> *your garden, or even your bathtub.*
> —ELISABETH KÜBLER-ROSS

> *I begin and end each day at my altar.*
> GURMUKH KAUR KHALSA

WALK INTO a room that is filled with the scent of lavender, diffused lighting, pastoral paintings, and the sounds of Miles Davis, and your mind will suddenly clear. Sit at a table in a fluorescent-lit kitchen with a pack of toddlers, the scent of cheeseburgers, and fingerprint-stained walls, and your mind will be a jumble of diverse thoughts, none of them calm.

The tradition of having a sacred space is rooted in ancient cultures, where an altar was a focal point of many homes. With our fast-paced and frenetic lives, more of us are trying to carve out a space for reflection and thought, be it a garage turned into a studio, a closet transformed into a meditation center, a bookshelf disguised as an altar, or a spot in the garden designated as a sanctuary. For the actress and jewelry designer Janet Gunn, that space is her converted garage, where the scents of fresh-cut roses and orange blossoms calm her. The actress Jenna von Oy finds solace in her guest room turned studio, where candles and lavender simultaneously stimulate and soothe her. The journalist Asha Blake's space is also a guest room, where late at night she burns candles and hand-tints photographs.

Gurmukh's Special Space

Gurmukh Kaur Khalsa, a yoga guru in Los Angeles whose studio has been frequented by Courtney Love, Cindy Crawford, Reese Witherspoon, and Madonna, helps many of her students attain peace in their lives by serving as a graceful example. Although high-powered celebrities and entertainment industry executives come to her to practice Kundalini yoga, they also take away sage advice on finding measures of balance, including ways to create a sacred space within their homes.

Gurmukh's sacred space is a converted cupboard, located near the front door of her Los Angeles home. She begins and ends each day at her altar, even if just for a moment. The shelf is covered with simple gifts from friends, greeting cards, rocks and shells, candles, photos of her daughter, and spiritual images. She asks her friends who travel to bring back a favorite stone or rock, which she proudly displays on her altar. She changes the altar often and counsels her students not to be afraid to change their spaces' contents regularly. Sometimes she adds an item that reminds her of someone from whom she is estranged, a sort of memento that draws that person of the past into her sphere.

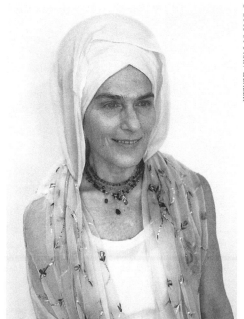

Gurmukh Kaur Khalsa

According to Gurmukh, your sacred space, at work or at home, should be wherever your eye is drawn. It should be clutter-free and have an element of yourself. For the Hole rocker Courtney Love's sacred space, she advised the addition of "singing bowls"—brass bowls that make a melodic singing sound. This allowed the recording artist's place for reflection to be accompanied by the meditative sounds of the bowls. For her student the producer Rick Rubin, who has helped mold the careers of musicians such as the Red Hot Chili Peppers, the sacred space is a music room. For all of her students, Gurmukh advocates "spring cleaning," getting rid of the excess so that the eye and the mind are able to rest, relax, and rejuvenate. Size does not matter, according to Gurmukh. In fact, the first altar she created, when she was four years old, was a shoe box with a candle.

Before Gurmukh moved into her new studio, Golden Bridge, she consulted a feng shui expert to create a space that would help the flow of energy and uplift the spirits of her students. The master, David Chow,

Gurmukh's Recipe for Your Own Sacred Space

Select a place where you will be able to have a measure of privacy; the purpose of the space is reflection.

Remember that size is not important.

Free the space of clutter, and keep it clean.

Include something that is living—a plant, herbs, or fresh flowers.

Choose colors that you like and respond to.

Include some fresh scents.

Energy needs to flow, so a nearby window is desirable.

Add candles with a scent that uplifts you. Go to a candle shop, select an assortment, and stay with the ones you really love.

Include remembrances from childhood, photographs, trinkets, and letters.

Add incense for its reputed power to alter the mind.

Select items that give you a feeling of universality, things that stimulate your creativity, and objects that help you "keep your heart open."

Remember that there are no hard-and-fast rules.

incorporated images of Gurmukh's own spiritual gurus, who have uplifted her spirit, into the space. The studio, with its gleaming oak floors and pristine white walls, glows from the many flickering candles and incense, which continuously emit both light and scent. Vases of fresh flowers, tapestries from India and Tibet, and bronze figures from Gurmukh's personal collection contribute to the soothing ambience.

Kelly Rutherford's Quiet Space

House hunting is a perfect opportunity to find your sacred space from among the rooms, nooks, and corners in hundreds of houses you will walk through in search of the one that is truly your home. When the *Melrose Place* actress Kelly Rutherford was hunting for her own place, she came upon the perfect bathroom and immediately knew that it was hers. She recalls, "When I saw it, I thought, I have to have this house!" Kelly's bathroom is a private and intimate space for herself. She always lights one of her several goddess aromatherapy candles. She says, "The key is to make your bathroom a spa for you. Create a sacred space in your house." In addition to her bathroom, Kelly's guest room is her "quiet space," home to a "really comfy chair. The light floods in just right from the windows." Kelly's sacred space allows her to enjoy "me-time" and feel lucky about the little details in life.

Tracee Ross's Happy Place

While some of us find serenity in spiritual sculptures and soothing scents, others prefer "out of the ordinary" objects that evoke feelings of whimsy. The *Girlfriends* actress Tracee Ross's happy place is her closet. She is a collector, so her closet is an eclectic gathering of colors and shapes that she can feast her eyes on. She explains, "I don't like drawers. I like to see everything. I figure, if you see it, you wear it." Her closet is filled with jewelry, scarves, bags, hats, shoes, feathers, and of course clothes, all in view. "It is like a vintage store!" Tracee exclaims. And it makes her happy.

Garcelle Beauvais-Nilon's Warm Haven

Like many, Garcelle Beauvais-Nilon relishes her bathtime; it's her time to take a breath and soak away her tensions. But more than the water itself, it is the atmosphere that this *NYPD Blue* actress immerses herself in. Her bathtub sits in a warm room with mustard-colored walls and Spanish tile details. A wooden cabinet is home to her array of beauty products, and the scent of fresh flowers fills the air. The bathroom is Garcelle's private space to indulge in simple, girlie pleasures. When she is ready for her evening bath, Garcelle dims the lights, takes out her gardenia-scented candle, adds a few drops of lavender essential oil to the soothing water, and periodically submerges below the steamy surface. Soon, her mind and body are relaxed as tensions float away.

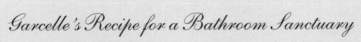

Garcelle's Recipe for a Bathroom Sanctuary

Mustard-colored walls

Spanish tile accents

Gardenia candles

Lavender essential oil

Beauty products in a wooden cabinet

Fresh flowers

Alter Your Energy with Feng Shui

Suddenly your neighbors paint their front door red and get rid of the doorbell, replacing it with wooden wind chimes. No, they aren't having a midlife crisis; more likely, they have been influenced by feng shui.

Feng shui, which literally means "wind and water," is an ancient Chinese system that helps people create harmony and the flow of positive energy, or *chi,* in their indoor and outdoor environments. Created thousands of years ago in rural China so that farmers could determine the most fruitful places to establish their homes, the art has captured the imaginations of many A-list Hollywood personalities. A feng shui home or office is strategically laid out—windows, doors, mirrors, and plants are placed according to beliefs that can effectually transform environments and ultimately change lives for the better. Accurate feng shui placement carefully balances each of the five elements, creating harmony. Here is a brief introduction to the five elements.

1. Fire
   Strength and assertion. Color: Red
   In decor, use fire elements such as candles and red fabric.

2. Earth
   Balance, organization, and practicality. Color: Yellow
   In decor, include soil in a potted plant and flower bed.

3. Metal
   Mental activity and thought processes. Colors: Silver and white
   In decor, use round objects that represent metal.

4. Water

Spirituality and meditation. Color: Black
In decor, use glass vases and clear marble stones.

5. Wood

Intuition, strong yet flexible. Color: Green
In decor, use live plants and anything that represents wood.

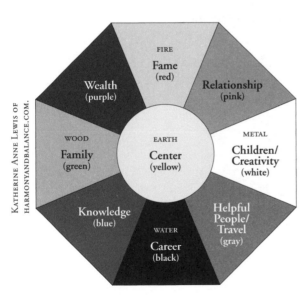

There are a few required elements in effective feng shui. First of all, you've got to have an open mind and trust that by painting your front door red (or burgundy or mauve), you are projecting power and authority. Next, you are going to need to get a hold of a bagua, the octagonal map or template that identifies the nine life areas. The bagua is placed over the main entrance to your home, usually with the career area at the front door. Last, you will need to be prepared to rearrange the innards of your entire house. Okay . . . you don't have to take feng shui to the extreme. If you add a candle here, a crystal there, and maybe a few plants, your life areas are also sure to benefit from the powers of feng shui.

Here is a brief introduction to the nine life areas:

1. Career
   Your involvement in the working world
   Color: Black

2. Helpful people
   Teachers, friends, and other methods by which luck enters
   Color: Gray

3. Children and creativity
   Key to personal, psychological, and spiritual growth
   Color: White

4. Relationships
   Both personal and professional
   Color: Pink

5. Fame
   Includes reputation and image
   Color: Red

6. Wealth
   In addition to financial prosperity, represents abundance
   Color: Purple

7. Family
   Both blood family and community of friends
   Color: Green

8. Knowledge
   Wisdom as well as new knowledge
   Color: Blue

9. Health
   At the center of the bagua, representing collective and individual health
   Color: Yellow

Katherine Anne Lewis's Everyday Feng Shui

Katherine Anne Lewis is a feng shui master and founder of Harmony and Balance. Before discovering the healing art of feng shui, she ran the accounting department of an entertainment company. While she enjoyed the work, the intensity soon weighed on her health, and she suffered an almost fatal bout of pneumonia. Something was clearly missing in her life. After she read a book on feng shui and applied some basic principles, her health improved and she fell in love with the practice. Intent on finding out all she could about this mysterious system that had saved her life, Katherine Anne birthed a new, much healthier career as a feng shui adviser. After studying the Tibetan Tantric Black Hat Sect method of feng shui more than seven years ago, she received her initial certification from an international certified Tibetan grand master.

By word of mouth, Katherine's practice quickly grew, and she now boasts a clientele of Oscar- and Emmy-award-winning actors, entertainment industry executives, the award-winning documentary filmmaker Binnur Karaevli, as well as corporations. Her new book, *Functional Feng*

Shui Remedies, helps readers create harmony in their work and play environments, be they bedrooms, hotel rooms, cars, or gardens. In addition, each chapter offers simple and economical feng shui remedies to improve wealth, relationships, careers, and health.

Not wanting to leave anything to chance, this past year several Oscar contenders consulted Katherine Anne as they eagerly awaited the results of balloting. They asked her to help with the areas in their homes that concerned reward and fortune. She advised them to shine lamps into the southern corners, which correspond to renown and fortune. She also recommended that they light three candles—for body, mind, and spirit—on a table in the southernmost areas of their homes to achieve fire in their areas of renown and recognition.

Feng shui is also used during the conception of shopping centers and office buildings. For The Grove, a 600,000-square-foot shopping mall in Los Angeles, the developers consulted Katherine Anne in the early stages of construction. She advised placing a large fountain, surrounded by flowers, lights, various colors, and music, as well as curved pathways throughout (straight lines are ill advised in feng shui). Jacaranda trees, which attract butterflies (believed to represent new beginnings, creativity, and life), were planted throughout, together with oak trees, which represent strength. The outdoor shopping center, which opened in 2002, has been wildly successful, no doubt due in part to the careful attention to principles of feng shui.

For the Downey Museum of Art in Downey, California, Katherine Anne recommended some simple changes to the buildings. An inviting sitting area with subtle lighting and a curved stone walkway leading to the entrance were added, and very likely influenced a doubling of the museum's yearly donations.

Katherine Anne believes that she is the bridge for her celebrity clients who need to cross over to new behavior and new ways of thinking in order to realize their goals. By making changes in their environment, they are able to take positive and concrete steps. They have more confidence, knowing that they have made these changes.

Feng shui is a process. Working with only two life areas at a time, Katherine Anne begins by extensively interviewing her clients. Recently, a well-known actress came to see Katherine Anne, lamenting a flagging career. As Katherine Anne walked through the actress's home, she noticed a large painting of water strategically placed within her fame and recognition area. What she needed was a painting with lots of red, the symbol of fire and fame. She replaced the painting with one that liberally used the color red and, for extra energy, backed it with red paper, unseen yet powerful. Katherine Anne's "cures" can be simple, anything from rearranging furniture to adding pots of water or plants and wind chimes. Katherine Anne says that the practice of feng shui, designed to bring harmony and balance and a semblance of sanity into everyone's life, is a bit like spring cleaning.

Katherine Anne's Recipe for More Positive Energy

Clear the Clutter to
    "Clear your mind
    Open your heart
    Receive your wishes" (SM)

Katherine Anne believes that celebrities seek out her services as a way to direct their lives through positive action. Adding this element of control helps relieve stress. Here are a few simple feng shui fix-its:

- I am woman, I am powerful.

Let the world know your strength by painting your front door red or a shade of red. The Chinese believe that red projects authority. Wear red shoes to a business meeting or, if you feel too conspicuous in red shoes, wear crimson undies.

- I'm looking for love.

Hang a wreath with pink flowers on your door and add planters placed in pairs along the path leading to the entrance. These let suitors know that your love light is definitely on.

- I'm still looking for love.

If you have mirrors in the bedroom that reflect on you and your partner in bed, remove them; they may signal that other people are interfering with your relationship.

- Show me the money.

If you measure your wealth in money, make certain that you have plenty of purple in your wealth area. Orchids also represent wealth. And if you feel that your money is flowing out, make certain you always keep your toilet seat closed. If it is left up, your money will just drain away.

- I'm dazed and confused.

Remember that a cluttered room equals a cluttered mind. Virtually every feng shui practitioner insists that chi will flow only through an un-cluttered space.

- I have a fever.

If you would like to have better health, add healthy plants to your health area.

- I can't sleep at night.

Eliminate clutter, including the junk under the bed as well as knick-knacks and photos on walls or dressers, and let the energy flow freely through the bedroom. Use soft colors like off-white or pale yellow, instead of stark white or bright colors. However, if your bedroom is also a place for romance, it's okay to have a bit of red in your relationship area.

- I still can't sleep at night.

Try placing a glass of water on a table level with your head, next to your bed. Don't drink the water, and it will absorb negative energy, making for a restful night.

- And baby makes three.

Make certain that a thorough clutter cleaning occurs before your new baby comes home. The baby's room should be filled with earth energy—pastel blue to calm, yellow for nourishment, and pale pink to gently stimulate.

• My teenager wants to paint it black.

Black is the color of introspection. If the thought of a room with black walls is beyond the pale for you, consider black furniture, electronics, or even a bedspread.

Katherine Anne's Recipe for a Romantic Feng Shui Bedroom

Remove all the stuff that you have stored under your bed. What lies under your bed is what feeds your body as you sleep, so make certain that you don't have any debris or residue of past loves.

Use your favorite soothing colors so that, as you walk in the door, you feel at ease. Warm earth colors encourage closeness, while a touch of red breeds passion.

Candles are great, as they ignite fire and passion.

Plants near the bed are fine; however, the leaves should be round.

Remove any mirrors that face the bed or are hung over the bed, as they invite trouble into a relationship.

Keep the relationship corner of the bedroom clean.

Hang a picture of you and your honey or add a pair of red candles (anything in pairs).

On the more extreme side, consider getting rid of that old mattress. There is nothing like starting anew.

Katherine Anne's Recipe for Better Business Through Feng Shui

Place your desk so that you look out (not with your back to the door). You want to be open to new opportunities and new clients.

Don't get rid of the family photographs on the desk, just set them to the side. The family is great for grounding; however, constantly looking at their photographs can interrupt the flow of work.

Ideally, the painting on the wall that is in your line of sight will include red, the color of passion and wealth. A simple solution for the lack of red is to back the painting with red paper.

Square or rectangular desks encourage making more money.

Remove the clutter. Holding on to old files, papers, and other junk keeps you living in the past.

Shannon Elizabeth's Feng Shui House

When friends, construction workers, repairmen, or anyone else enters your home, they leave a little bit of themselves there. The actress Shannon Elizabeth's personal life is quite different from the life she portrays in *American Pie, American Pie 2, Jay and Silent Bob Strike Back,* and *Scary Movie.* Shannon leads a very spiritual life. She explains, "I have my house feng shuied a couple of times a year because energies change with

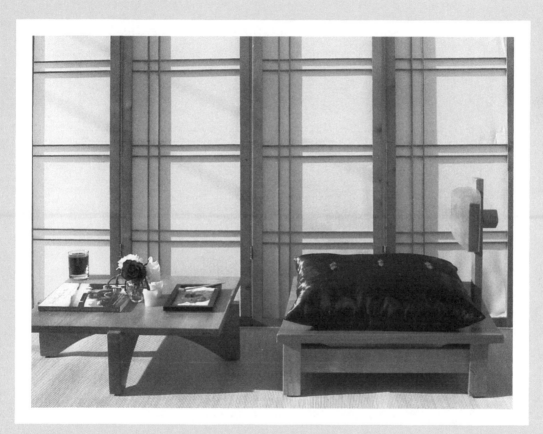

Laurel's indoor meditative space.

Shannon's Recipe for a Feng Shui Meditation Room

Lots of windows and glass doors, allowing in a flood of natural light

A wooden piece with a God statue built into it and a bench for candles and incense

Mini Moroccan rug

3 pillows

Incense

Candles

3 Buddhas

3 Ganeshes

Seasonal feng shui energy clearing

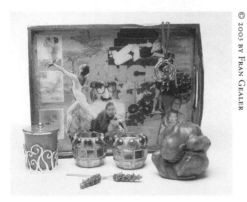

Small sacred space.

© 2003 BY FRAN GEALER

the seasons. My husband [also an actor] and I share a meditation room. It is also the location in our home that is strong for prosperity, so it is a place for achievement awards too. We try to keep the room just for us, since when other people come into your space, they leave their own energy."

Shannon's meditation room is filled with gifts, mementos, and spiritual statues that help to ground her. She says, "We have a wooden piece with a God statue built into it and a bench that we place candles and incense on. It was given to us by our contractor and his girlfriend. We use it as a centerpiece. We have a mini

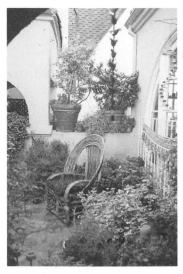

Sacred space in Gurmukh's garden.

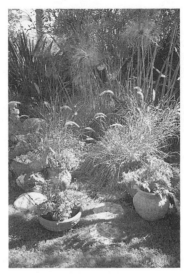

Sharon's garden.

Moroccan rug, lots of pillows, incense, candles, Buddhas, and Ganeshes. We try to keep everything in threes. It is a feng shui thing. The room is filled with beautiful light from the windows and glass doors, and we have a cool lamp that lets off this great light. But usually when I meditate at night, I just light candles."

RESOURCES

www.harmonyandbalance.com
Functional Feng Shui Remedies by Katherine Anne Lewis
The Everything Feng Shui Book by Katina Z. Jones
Feng Shui in 10 Simple Lessons by Jane Butler-Biggs
Feng Shui: The Art of Living by Rosalind Simmons

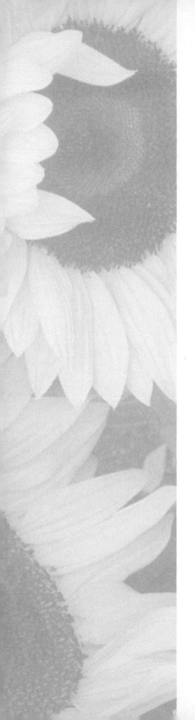

Chapter Twelve

Work Out Your Body, Work Out Your Mind

When I walk, my entire body is working at
the same time and I am physically balanced.
—*ALFRE WOODARD*

OUR CULTURE has become so engrossed by the physicality of fitness that we often neglect to recognize its emotional and mental benefits. More than a mode to attain a toned physique and bulging muscles, excerise has been recognized as one of the most efficient methods of stress reduction and inner balance. It can improve your mood and brighten your day while also promoting a good night's sleep.

Many of us unknowingly experience the stress-reducing benefits of exercise on a daily basis. Those of you who hit the gym or go for a jog after a hard day at the office know what I'm talking about. Fitness can be the best way to escape from the daily grind. Whether you are more inclined to dance, spin, hike, Rollerblade, do tai chi, or weight-train, you can find an emotional release from either an intense, muscle-trembling, sweat-producing workout or a light workout that elevates your heart rate. Regular physical activity is proven to boost self-esteem because it promotes weight loss, increased muscle tone, personal achievement, a feeling of control over your life and body, increased social interaction or, on the contrary, enjoyment of personal time and improved physical functioning. Chemically, exercise can promote the production of endorphins, brain chemicals that can elevate your mood (i.e., give you a "runner's high"). Additionally, running, biking, or hiking in fresh air under the warm sun has even been purported to be a natural antidepressant. The fact is that our bodies are meant to move, so move that body of yours!

Dance Your Stress Away

While some people are turned off of physical fitness because of expensive gym memberships, equipment, and accessories; having to fight traffic to go to the gym; and dealing with sweaty equipment and creepy voyeurs, exercise doesn't have to be so cumbersome. Greg Isaacs, owner of Greg Isaacs 360 gym in Los Angeles and a celebrity trainer to such A-listers as Pierce Brosnan, Goldie Hawn, and several members of the cast of *Friends,* is certainly familiar with pumping iron, running for miles on end, and spinning until it feels as though your legs just might fall off, yet he believes that "dance is the perfect integration of mind, body, and spirit because it is a natural movement of the body. It is a nonjudgmental, nonspecific form of fitness that exercises you entirely. For those of you who are in search of a mind-body connection, simply free your body and dance. Turn on your favorite song and feel the groove. Let your body sway until you feel the music inside of you, in your mind, body, and soul. Allow the music to move you both mentally and physically." Dance does more than liberate the mind; it is a release for the body and an unbelievably efficient workout that tones, tightens, and destresses. Don't forget the age-old adage that the dancer's body is the "perfect" body.

While it is easy to find that one workout you love and repeat it night after night, week after week, repetition can cause boredom and increase the likelihood that you will quit working out altogether. Also, it is important to change it up a bit because you need to make sure to exercise all the muscles of your body in different ways or risk hitting a plateau, or diminishing returns. Try to find at least two types of exercise that you love and switch off every other day. Cross training is a great option for those who bore easily because it incorporates various types of physical activity within one workout, producing the quickest and most lasting results. Think of exercise as an endless array of options, all of which you need to try before settling down with your selection. Consulting a well-rounded and well-educated fitness expert is a great first step on the path to determining your fitness favorites.

Many celebrities work out with personal trainers to keep their fitness programs fresh, fun, and effective. Trainers also help keep you motivated. If the last thing you want to do when you roll out of bed in the morning is exercise, knowing that someone is waiting for you at the gym, park, or outside your front door will surely help to get your body moving.

Melissa Rivers Relaxes with Her Baby

While E!'s Melissa Rivers certainly puts in her share of hours at the gym, she also enjoys exercising on her own time, with her son in tow. She says, "My son loves the beach, and I love being with my son. So instead of de-stressing alone, I do it with him. We head down to the bike path on the beach, I put him in the Baby Jogger, and I Rollerblade behind him. It gives me a mini workout, gets my blood flowing, and allows me to spend some quality time with my son. He loves it. We have done this together since he was an infant. It is quiet time for both of us."

Carnie Wilson and Cardio Barre

Carnie Wilson credits Cardio Barre with "completely changing my life." One third of the Wilson Phillips singing trio, Carnie was known as much for her size as for her vocal talent. She discovered Richard Giorla and Cardio Barre after undergoing a highly publicized and controversial gastric bypass surgery that drastically reduced her size but left her with sagging skin.

Developed by Richard, a former New York dancer, the no-impact, ballet-based Cardio Barre helps develop long, lean muscles by using the

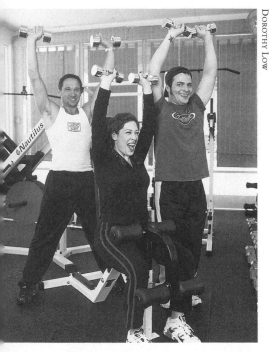

DOROTHY LOW

Richard Giorla (left) of Cardio Barre with Carnie Wilson (seated).

same ballet barre that dancers train with. Holding on to the barre, students isolate small muscle groups and learn how to focus and concentrate. This fun, fast-paced, fat-burning, sweat-dripping, muscle-toning class combines strength training and stretching while providing an intense cardio workout. Carnie, the actress Amanda Pays, the singer Nikki Costa, Amy Davidson from the television series *8 Simple Rules for Dating My Teenage Daughter,* and Jennie Garth from *Beverly Hills 90210* are just a handful of Richard's celebrity clients who work it, feel it, and keep coming back for more.

While they have "celebrity schedules," Richard doesn't let their minds drift. He explains, "I keep them in focus. Because of the high repetitions, the hour goes by quickly." While all exercise programs help you destress, Cardio Barre is different because "you are always lifting your chest and chin up, working in a proud and confident stance." Richard's students walk out of the studio with their chests open, shoulders back, and heads held high. In fact, students find that just about everything from confidence and mood to chests and butts is raised in Richard's classes. Carnie found that "after one month, my butt was actually higher . . . it was lifted. The class made me feel my endorphins for the first time. I feel positive and hopeful, no longer like a lazy pig." When she doesn't work out, Carnie says she "feels depressed." It's amazing what a few weights and leg lifts (along with a great trainer) can do for your body and self-esteem.

Richard says it is this sense of accomplishment, the instant results and the positive reinforcement, that draws celebrities and ordinary people alike to his class. His energy forces his students to concentrate and be "in the zone," a euphoria that he hopes they continue to feel throughout the day.

Cardio Kitchen

You can easily re-create Cardio Barre moves in the privacy of your home, using a countertop, the back of a sturdy chair, or a high work surface as your barre. Here are three easy exercises that can help trim and tone your body into what is considered by many to be the epitome of physique—the dancer's body!

Richard's Recipe for Perfectly Lifted Buttocks and Glutes

This exercise is guaranteed to lift your butt if you do it at least 3 times a week.

Facing the "barre," place both hands parallel on top of the barre at a comfortable distance apart.

With your left toes facing the barre, flex and turn out the right foot so that your feet are perpendicular to each other.

Keeping your legs straight, lift your right leg directly behind you as high as is comfortable.

Do 50 to 100 repetitions without touching the foot to the floor.

Lower and repeat with the other leg.

Richard's Recipe for Shapely Calves

This exercise can be done anywhere. It doesn't require a chair or countertop. Each position works a different part of the calf.

For the inner calf, place heels together with feet turned out, creating the shape of a V.

Keeping your legs straight, lift both heels off the floor, then return them to the floor.

Repeat 50 times.

For the center calf, place feet parallel, 6 to 8 inches apart.

Lift both heels, then return them to the floor.

Repeat 50 times.

For the outer calf, turn feet inward, with the toes facing each other, creating an inverted V.

Lift both heels, then return them to the floor.

Repeat 50 times.

Richard's Recipe for Sexy Legs and Butt

Doing this exercise will work the inner thighs, buttocks, quadriceps, ankles, and calves.

Place your body alongside a chair or countertop as "barre."

Hold the barre with the hand closest to it.

Open your legs wider than shoulder width and turn your feet outward.

Make certain that your knees are over your toes when you bend your legs at the knees.

Hold your body upright with shoulders back, stomach in, and chest lifted.

Make certain your pelvis is in alignment (don't stick your butt out) so that you are working with a straight spine.

Bend your knees as you lower yourself straight down to knee level, so that your thighs are parallel to the floor and perpendicular to your calves.

Return to a standing position using fluid movement. (This is a classic ballet move.)

On the way up, be certain to squeeze your inner thighs and buttocks.

Repeat 50 times.

For a more advanced workout, repeat the sequence on your toes.

Richard has created a series of Cardio Barre videos that are available by visiting his Web site, www.cardiobarre.com.

Kathy Kaehler's Celebrity Circuit Walk

Kathy Kaehler, "fitness trainer to the stars" and the *Today* show's exercise correspondent recommends walking as one of the easiest and most enjoyable, stress-reducing, and effective workouts. Fortunately, more than serving as a means of transportation, walking is a safe and low-impact way to a toned and healthy body. Your excuse that you don't want to join a gym because it's too crowded, too expensive, and too far won't work anymore as your get-out-of-exercise-free card. No gym is required to walk, and no special equipment is needed (except a good pair of shoes). You can walk virtually anywhere, for any amount of time, and you can do it for free! You can choose to stroll, walk briskly, speed-walk, or maybe even jog or run. Walking is an activity that you can do with a partner, in a group, or alone. The options are endless.

Even celebrities enjoy long walks. In fact, Kathy incorporates walking into the fitness routines of several of her celebrity clients, including Julia Roberts, Nancy Travis, and Alfre Woodard. Kathy loves walking because, she explains, "It has been proven to be effective for weight loss. It keeps you in the aerobic zone, it's easy on the joints and effective at shaping and toning." Since she is a personal trainer, she must keep her clients motivated by keeping the exercises fun and interesting, so Kathy often turns a simple walk into a challenging fitness routine. She says, "You can make walking more challenging by adding stairs or tying a jump rope around your waist and stopping to jump rope at intervals." Soon you will find that you have created a highly effective and incredibly exhausting circuit-training workout.

While walking is an activity that most of us are quite accustomed to, a few guidelines may make your "new" fitness routine a bit more effective. First of all, the surgeon general recommends moderate amounts of activities, such as a brisk walk, at least thirty minutes per day for overall health. It doesn't really matter what you are doing with your arms—hanging them by your sides, swinging them freely, or assuming the speed-walking position of bent arms and fisted hands, though the speed-walk position is the best way to ensure that your heart rate is increasing. Proper position being

Kathy's Celebrity Circuit Walk

Get in your car and mark off ¼, ½, ¾, and 1 mile.

Return to your starting point and put your running shoes on.

Walk the first ¼ mile; stop and jump rope for 200 revolutions.

Run to the ½-mile point; stop and do 20 squats or lunges.

Run to the ¾-mile point; stop and do 200 jump rope revolutions.

Fast-walk to the end.

This variety will keep up your interest. If your heart rate has a chance to go up and down, you will get into shape more quickly. This type of speed adjustment is also great for the treadmill, on which you would start the circuit at 1 mile and gradually build up to 3 miles.

Try to do this 4 to 6 times each week.

your arms bent at a 90-degree angle. Allow your arms to swing freely so that they come up to about chest level. Keep your fingers curled into loose fists. And move your feet at a brisk pace. Kathy also recommends a certain type of shoe: "I like to feel overall support with cushion in the heel and flexibility in the sole, so when push off, I feel supported." Remember that all feet are shaped slightly differently, so be sure that your shoe correctly molds to *your* foot. Now you are ready to get walking!

Like many celebrities, Kathy lives in Los Angeles and has the opportunity to take long walks down the beach with her clients. The ocean offers an incredibly healing and calming environment; the water brings a sense of serenity that can be challenging to achieve in a gym or on busy streets.

In addition to being a relaxing environment, the beach offers an unstable surface (the sand), which forces your body to work a little harder to stabilize, thereby gaining coordination along with strength. Other celebrities prefer to walk in the hills or on hiking trails. Similarly serene, mountains and hills provide a strenuous terrain filled with inclines and declines. One well-known entertainer enjoys taking walks in her neighborhood, which imparts a sense of security and familiarity, whereas the beach or the mountains can yield a sense of escape.

Alfre Woodard's Fitness Walk

Walking, for the Oscar-nominated actress Alfre Woodard, is "empowering." Alfre walks with Kathy, her fitness "guru." "When I walk," she says, "my entire body is working at the same time and I am physically balanced." It is the element of "being in charge" that Alfre loves about walking. In addition to the obvious physical benefits, walking "helps me take control of my own thoughts," states the actress who is known for her roles in *Passion Fish, Love & Basketball, Miss Ever's Boys,* for which she won an Emmy and a Golden Globe. Alfre refers to the ability to control her thoughts as "what we call 'sane.' "

Alfre credits Kathy with helping her train herself back into her childhood mind-set, when exercise was intuitive and organic. An athlete and a Girl Scout for ten years, Alfre likes nothing better than a hike. For her, being outdoors and not in the gym is essential. Wherever she is, from the country roads of New England to the beaches of California, she walks. She fondly remembers her introduction to walking as exercise nineteen years ago while making a movie in Zimbabwe. The locals thought she was crazy as she strode along the road, "walking for exercise."

While she enjoys the restorative benefits of walking, Alfre also takes pleasure in the fact that its toning and slimming benefits come with minimal effort. This ease is important to Alfre, who says, "When I set off on a walk, I need nothing to start. I just put one foot in front of the other." Still, she does have two simple rules that she tries to follow:

1. Never walk with your cell phone. It would be like sitting in church and talking with your friends.
2. Never walk with people who gossip. It defeats the purpose of relaxing into a meditative state.

Kathy makes Alfre's walk interesting by incorporating various types of activities into it. Sometimes, Alfre and Kathy walk for a quarter mile, find a bench and do squats, then walk another quarter mile, and end the workout with sprints at the local tennis court. Alfre has established her own circuit training routine through the neighborhood, which keeps her interested and determined not to give up.

Kathy herself walks to reduce stress and maintain her serenity. Walking takes her out of the frenetic environment of her kids, husband, housekeeper, clients, magazines, television appearances, and everything else that goes along with her life. It allows Kathy time to think, plan, and get a better perspective on life. She has even created her own "Twenty-one Mile-a-Week Club," with the goal of walking twenty-one miles each week. Sometimes she's successful, and sometimes she isn't. Either way, she says, "I don't beat myself up over it." Setting a goal like Kathy's is a great way to work out and a reason to get out of bed in the morning or take the long way when walking to lunch.

Alicia Leigh Willis Punches Out Her Frustrations

Sometimes it takes more than a few deep breaths and contorted poses to achieve inner peace. While the *General Hospital* star Alicia Leigh Willis loves to do yoga, she says that boxing is her favorite destressor: "It is such a hard workout. When you get in the ring and spar, it takes a lot of endurance. But when you are done, you are buzzing. Your endorphins kick in and you feel so good. It is a great way to release frustrations. Plus, when you get in shape, you feel better. When I don't work out, I feel dull."

Gunnar Peterson's Life-Altering Exercise

"Fitness is something that you do for yourself now and for everyone else later." The celebrity personal trainer Gunnar Peterson is a firm believer that exercise does more than just benefit the body today. He believes that exercise has the ability to positively affect tomorrow, years, and even decades from now. When you exercise, your endorphins are pumping, your blood is flowing, and your body is changing. In turn, your self-esteem is enhanced, your mood is elevated, and you are kinder to those around you. These results are all reinforced by studies and statistics. The naturally occurring relationship between mood and exercise affects most everyone, including Gunnar, who exercises for a living. He declares, "I know that I

act differently after a good workout." Gunnar says, "I have a couple of petite female clients who hit the punching bag and say 'Wow, that feels so
good!' It is because they are releasing excess energy, essentially, letting off
some steam, resulting in destressing."

While it may feel good for some of us, others have to force themselves
into the gym every day. But the fact is that exercise is not suddenly going
to get easy. Nor will it go away. "Since you know that you have got to do
it, you may as well love it," says Gunnar. "Or at least like it. What is the alternative? Forfeit your quality of life? No!" If exercise is drudgery for you,
then try to change your perspective on it. Says Gunnar, "I don't know how
many times I have repeated this statement to my clients, but if you get
yourself to enjoy the process of exercise, the whole experience is better,
and you benefit that much more." So, if you love swinging a tennis racket,
hitting a golf ball, braving a hiking trail, or dancing the night away, you
are getting a great workout— and look at that, you even have a smile on
your face!

Gunnar's celebrity clientele has included many of the top A-listers, such
as Angelina Jolie, Jennifer Lopez, Ben Affleck, Jennifer Connelly, Amber
Valletta, Tracee Ross, Sylvester Stallone, Cameron Diaz, Penélope Cruz,
and Michelle Branch. But the fact that they are celebrities doesn't mean he
is any easier on them. Anyone who works out with Gunnar has an unpar-
alleled gym experience. His five-thousand-square-foot Beverly Hills facility is ultraprivate, immaculately clean, and filled with so many equipment
options that it includes multiple rooms, six flights of outdoor stairs, a basketball and tennis court, rock-climbing wall, putting green, and personal
changing area. Even with all of this, Gunnar allows only two clients, receiving one-on-one training, at any one time in his facility. Celebrities, as

well as anyone else who can afford his personal training, are used to living the high life, and Gunnar is sensitive to that fact. "These are people who have front-row seats and backstage passes to life. I want their gym experience to be on par. They still are working, sweating, grinding, and feeling the pain, but where I can offer ease, why wouldn't I?"

The ease is in the ambience as well as in the quality and constant variation of the workout. While Gunnar certainly works his clients, he does so with minimal injury. "Some other trainers take pride in kicking their clients' butts. Why? I want my clients to be able to walk in the morning." Unfortunately, the older you get, the harder it is to get those tight joints and weak muscles moving. Gunnar says, "I remember one day Cameron [Diaz] and Stallone [Sylvester] were in here at the same time. Cameron commented on how her workout was so hard, but good. Stallone looked over and said, 'Yeah, just wait to see how it feels in thirty years!' Stallone has never missed a workout. He has been regularly coming in here, filled with energy, always in a good mood, never late, and he works out like it counts, every rep. He is incredibly focused."

Gunnar declares, "We have all heard the age-old adage 'If you don't use it, you lose it,' and we know it applies, so do it. Move it!" The problem often is that we feel almost immortal, like nothing is going to happen to us, regardless of how we take care of our bodies. That is until reality smacks us in the face with the sudden death of a friend or family member and we find ourselves reevaluating our own lifestyles and thinking about the consequences of our choices. Immediately, we jump-start our healthy food and exercise regimens. We fill our refrigerators with whole grains, fruits, vegetables, and low-fat foods. We reinstate our gym memberships and somehow find the time to jump on the treadmill or hit the bag three times a week. Unfortunately, the severity of reality begins to fade, and we start to slack off. Suddenly, our days are too full to exercise, and we stop at fast-food drive-throughs in a desperate attempt to throw some sort of nourishment down our throats. We are back to the grind and waiting for another reality-jolting reminder of just how precious and fragile life is. Well, stop waiting for something drastic to happen and start working out right now. You will be in a better mood today, less stressed tomorrow, and healthier and happier in the long run.

Amber Valletta's Tension Tamer

The supermodel Amber Valletta's svelte figure doesn't just magically appear. She has to work to obtain such perfection. Gunnar pushes her to work it three times a week at his private gym. And as she tones and tightens, her mind releases a bit of pent-up tension, allowing her to walk out lighter in both body and mind. "I feel great when I sweat and get the toxins out," says Amber, "and I like to see my muscles working when I box. Sometimes, I just beat up that bag. By nature, I am a competitive person." Gunnar constantly changes up her exercise routine, throwing in weights, core training, jumping, boxing, and kickboxing. Regardless of the type of exercise, she makes

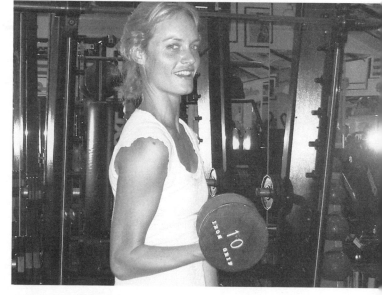

Amber Valletta flexing her muscles.

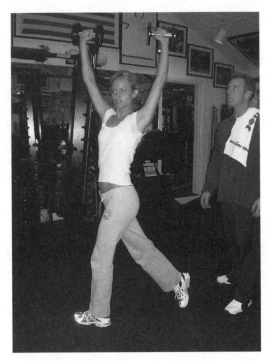

sure that she is having fun while still working hard. When not in the gym, Amber loves hiking in the Santa Monica Mountains. It is her time to get away from all the commotion in the city, breathe fresh air, and move her body.

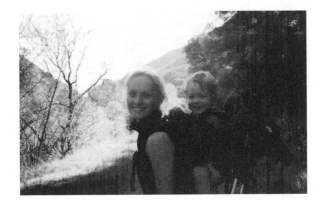

Amber Valletta working out with trainer Gunnar Peterson.

Amber Valletta hiking with her son.

Mari Winsor's Pilates

Mari Winsor is one of the best-known Pilates mavens in the United States. She teaches just about every A-list celeb, including Daisy Fuentes, Dustin Hoffman, Sharon Stone, Melanie Griffith, Drew Barrymore, Meg Ryan, Jamie Lee Curtis, Jewel, and Minnie Driver, how to "use their power-house" and gain strength, length, and flexibility. She also has several videos, which you may have seen through her many infomercials. So why have so many celebrities gravitated to her to get their abs, buns, and thighs in shape? "Because it works!" exclaims Mari. "My Pilates is dynamic. Other classes aren't dynamic enough. You aren't going to change your body unless you move it. And in my classes, you move it a lot!" Mari learned the art of Pilates from Romana Kryzanowska, who was a protégée of Pilates himself. Talk about a lineage of masters!

While Pilates sculpts the body, it also destresses. Mari explains, "Exercise is probably the best natural destressor there is because you clear your mind. We get stressed out when we have too much going on, too much on our minds, and we feel as though we have no time. Working out makes us clear our minds, especially with Pilates, because you have to do the precise movements correctly in order to benefit." Pilates can change more than your body; it can change your life. "Melanie Griffith gave me a quote that I put in my book. She said, 'It changed my life.' And it really can," Mari admits.

So what does Mari do to stay mentally serene and physically sculpted? Pilates and a ballet class three times a week. She says, "Teaching, for me, is a great destressor. I love to teach. I love to watch the changes in people, the revelations, the results!"

Susan Lucci's At-Home Exercise Routine

To keep that petite Erica Kane body of hers, the actress Susan Lucci does Pilates. She explains, "Every morning, I stretch before even getting out of bed. My favorite exercise is Pilates. I have been doing it for six years now.

Once I get out of bed, I do twenty to thirty minutes of mat Pilates. I also do push-ups, crunches, and different exercises to increase agility. Sometimes, I just bounce on my ball. It is important to have fun while you're working out." Susan has the Mari Winsor Pilates tapes, which are a great way to get in your workout without leaving home. She explains, "When I am too busy for traditional workouts, I try to fit exercise into my life by taking the stairs instead of the elevator and parking on the far side of a parking lot."

Holistic Fitness

Exercise can definitely destress. But more than that, according to the celebrity personal trainer Gregory Joujon-Roche, exercise can help to develop your sense of self. He says, "If I start my day with 'me-time,' I am more productive, creative, giving, and patient. It sets the tone for my day's experience." Sometimes all you need is ten minutes, and sometimes you need two hours, but whatever it is, dedicate a portion of your day to yourself. Says Gregory, "It depends on where my energy level is. Sometimes, all I need to do is walk on the treadmill and *breathe*. It is similar to how I train my clients. Every session is different because it all depends on the awareness of that moment and what serves the client best for the session." Well, Gregory is clearly doing something right considering that his company, Holistic Fitness, is known for turning actors into superheroes, everyday folk into rock stars, and showing top executives where their true power lies. His clients have included Brad Pitt in preparation for *Troy*, PINK for her new album and world tour, Pierce Brosnan in preparation for *Die Another Day,* model Gisele in order to keep that Victoria's Secret body in shape, Tobey Maguire for *Spiderman,* Julianna Margulies for *Ghost Ship,* Demi Moore for *Striptease* and *GI Jane,* as well as Gwen Stefani, Rachel Weisz, and James Franco to name a few. Greg's been around the world with the Spice Girls and even met with Richard Branson and the Sultan of Brunei.

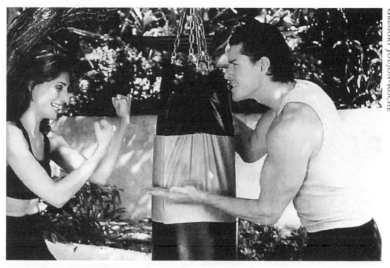

Gregory Joujon-Roche of Holistic Fitness with actress Jo Champa.

Gregory clearly has the know-how to transform regular bodies into superherolike figures, but how does this relate to the mind? He helps to redirect the reasons for working out. While he maintains emphasis on intense training and corrective exercise, he also works on strengthening the essence and presence of who we are. "We need to own who we are, step up, take notice, and breathe into the being we radiate to the world. Many people are so goal oriented and driven by false perceptions. They have this image of where they want their bodies to be—how thin, muscular, lean, or ripped. I try to provide a different perspective as it pertains to fitness, thus a different experience every time. I want my clients to take a little responsibility for his or her training. It's a give and take experience, a shared collaboration, not the Guru Greg show, how boring and un-evolving. Let's do it together. I provide the information and motiva-

Got 2 Hours?

If you have 2 hours to dedicate to exercise, Greg suggests that you start slowly and work up.

Begin with cardio. Jump on a treadmill, take a walk around the block, or go for a bike ride.

After the cardio, take some time to stretch.

Gregory suggests concentrating on one or two body parts per day.

tion then step back and watch my clients experience and work out the process for themselves. In the end they don't need a trainer, they got themselves in shape and that's the magic."

Holistic Fitness is the one-stop shop in Hollywood for fitness. Greg works with the finest fitness experts, doctors, and nutritionists in the world. "We are a company of about thirty specialists, all congruent in the Holistic philosophy of fitness, and overall well-being, including martial arts, gymnastics, yoga, personal training, massage, and nutrition." Recently, Greg teamed up with the top stunt coordinators and action experts in the business to create XL Action Team. Together they share more than two thousand film credits and actors from Tom Cruise to Lucy Liu and are taking Hollywood by storm. "When signing new clients, I begin by asking lots of questions to find out what his or her goals are, and how they want to get there. I try to keep the process interesting and creative, from the types of workouts to the food served. Hey, when in doubt go surfing. There's nothing like nature to bring out your true personality."

Got 10 Minutes?

Gregory says that how to spend your 10 minutes really depends on your state of mind.

If you are in need of a blast of energy, power up your body with cardio. It gets the blood moving.

If you've got too much going on in your head, then take those 10 minutes to breathe, refocus, and stretch.

"Spice Girl" Mel C Finds Her Identity Through Fitness

Melanie Chisholm of the Spice Girls sought out Gregory's help when she found herself sapped of energy and questioning her identity. The solution was a mind-and-body-focused fitness and nutrition plan that fit into the singer's lifestyle. Gregory and Mel C created the regimen together, based on her needs at the moment, as well as her likes and dislikes. For Mel C, Holistic Fitness was a life-altering experience. She says, "Holistic Fitness helped me get in touch with my body and [establish] a connection between mind, body, and spirit." She says that she realized, "you must begin where you are. Love yourself right here and now and then move forward. I realized that fitness is an inner journey that I create—no one else does. To be emotionally exposed to the world of entertainment and all that lives there, so much is required of me, which means I need an incredible amount of inner strength, peace, and stability."

RESOURCES

www.gregisaacs360.com
www.cardiobarre.com
www.winsorpilates.com
Pilates Power House by Mari Winsor
www.holisticfitness.com

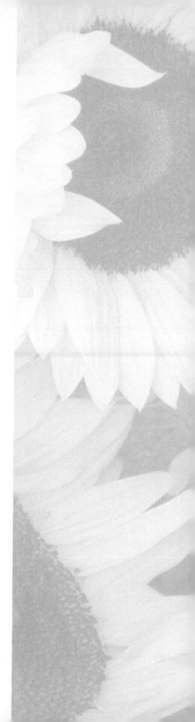

Chapter Thirteen

Little Luxuries

To me [catnaps], that is a real luxury.
—AMBER VALLETTA

SOME OF US feel so overextended that even ten minutes a day dedicated to our serenity seems like a splurge. We hope that after reading this book you will find a way to insert a few serenity savers into your juggling act. At least for now, add some little luxuries to your day that require no extra time or preparation; simply sneak them into your routine.

Hair Conditioner

My (Laurel) personal favorite little luxury? Hair conditioner. I love thick, creamy conditioner that leaves my hair so smooth I hardly need a brush. Yes, conditioner of this caliber does cost a few dollars more than the average grocery store brand, but every morning as I stand in the shower gliding my fingers through knotless strands of hair, I smile. In fact, my morning routine is shortened by about five minutes by avoiding the painstaking repetition of pulling my brush through knots and tangles, allowing me to enjoy a few moments each morning to do something for myself before rushing off to my daily grind.

Conditioner doesn't catch your fancy? Here are some other suggestions for little luxuries:

- What about cozy pajamas made of the silkiest silk or thick flannel pajamas that call out for cuddling?
- To ease those tired feet after a long high-heeled day, you can slather on tingling eucalyptus or peppermint foot cream like Origins Step Lively energizing foot cream. The simple scent of lavender, whether in the pure form of a living sprig growing in your window planter, an essential oil, a candle, or a sachet, has been proven to promote relaxation. I carry a small vial of lavender essential oil in my purse so that as I run between meetings or before I hop on an airplane I can smell the ease-inducing fragrance.
- When you hear a funny phrase or see a silly image that reminds you of your husband or boyfriend, it is hard not to smile. Carry around a card, a note on a napkin, or an e-mail from your love and pull it out in moments of

misery and stress. Tuck a photo of your daughter or a silly image of a kissing fish that curves your lips into a smile into an office drawer.

- Delete that annoying flying saucer that zips across your computer screen when not in use and replace it with a more soothing screen saver, like photos of your family and friends. You can even create a slide show displaying images of your wedding, your dog, or that fabulous kiss with your husband under the mistletoe that was caught on camera last Christmas.
- When you are walking down the street and you hear a bird chirping, don't ignore it. Look up into the trees, the sky, or along a telephone wire and try to find the exact bird singing you that song.
- Allow yourself to be silly—dress up your nails with blue glitter polish (if you can get away with it at work) or laugh out loud instead of keeping it down to a chuckle. Life shouldn't always be taken so seriously. If you allow yourself to live, you will . . . with a smile.

Amber Valletta's Personal Pleasures

The supermodel Amber Valletta takes pleasure in her son, especially when he is happy. "When my son is in a good mood," she says, "that is a great destressor. Nothing else brings me such joy!" When she has a few extra moments, she takes catnaps. "To me, that is a real luxury," she says. "I also love to read and go to the movies. It is great escapism." But when Amber goes out on the town, she shakes all the tension out of her body. "I like to dance," she declares. "If I am out somewhere at a club, every once in a while I will just go crazy and dance for hours until I break a sweat."

Kelly Rutherford Unboggles Her Mind

Bills have the tendency to pile up to the point that the stack resembles the Leaning Tower of Pisa. Then it is time to take control of the mind-boggling mound. To make the whole process a bit less stressful, do what the actress Kelly Rutherford does—play music.

"Sometimes," Kelly admits, "my American Express bill calls for something calming. So I turn on some classical music, sit down, light a candle, and then open the bill and see what is inside." When bills aren't the source of her stress, but life in general seems to be weighing on Kelly's shoulders, she turns the lights out early. She explains, "When I am really stressed, sometimes I come home, have an early dinner, and get to bed by nine. I end up having the most amazing night's sleep, and I wake up in the morning feeling refreshed."

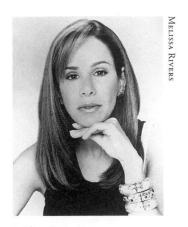

MELISSA RIVERS

Melissa Rivers

Melissa Rivers Carves Out "Me-Time"

Balancing television shows, fashion reviews, and her family, Melissa Rivers has figured out a way to carve out a little "me-time" so she can unwind and put herself back in balance. The moment she walks in the door of her home, Melissa removes all of her jewelry. "Taking off my jewelry signals that the day is over and I am home." Once she is settled, Melissa finds solace in her aromatherapy candles, which she keeps all around the house. Her candles provide a soothing atmosphere, unlike the spotlights and cameras of a television set. Late at night, after she puts her baby to bed, she lights a candle and finishes her evening activities. The flickering light and soothing scent allow her mind to calm as she begins to decompress and prepare for a relaxing night, releasing the stresses of the day.

Tracee Ross Flips

The actress Tracee Ross is a big fan of magazine flipping as a "me-time" activity. She says, "I buy a stack of magazines and flip through them. I rarely read them. I read books, but I flip through magazines. I pull out sheets of clothes I like, and I use the clothing pictures for *Girlfriends* to design my outfits for the show."

Lauren Holly Breathes

When the actress Lauren Holly has less than five minutes to destress and rebalance, she looks to her kids or her dog, whichever is available at that needed moment. "They will lie right on top of me. My son is just starting to talk, and he says, 'Ma loves to talk about the day!' That is what we do. He lies on my stomach and we talk about the day. I stroke his arm, and it is so relaxing!" When she doesn't have even five minutes to spare, she resorts to deep breathing. Many people do not know how or often forget to breathe. Rather than taking deep, cleansing breaths, many of us take short and shallow breaths and wonder why we feel so fatigued. Lauren admits that she is guilty of this too. "But then you finally take a deep, relaxing breath, and it feels so good!"

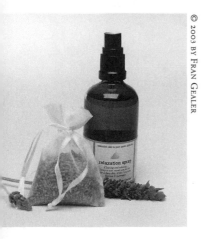

Garcelle Beauvais-Nilon Spritzes

Garcelle Beauvais-Nilon tries to make destressing a constant in her daily life. Whether she is at home relaxing, driving in traffic, or hard at work on the set of *NYPD Blue,* she is sure to incorporate at least one relaxing ritual into each day. Like many of us, Garcelle spends plenty of time in the car. Instead of getting frustrated when stuck in a traffic jam, she cleanses the air of unhealthy exhaust and allows herself a momentary break through the simple spritz of her handy lavender essential oil spray. She says, "Since we spend so much time in the car, we should try to enjoy it. Lavender always puts my mind at ease."

Susan Lucci Likes Warm Lemon Water

There is something soothing about sipping a warm drink to begin and end your day. For the *All My Children* star Susan Lucci, that drink is a warm glass of water with a squeeze of lemon. She explains, "I am trying to cut down on my coffee intake, because too much caffeine can be dehydrating. Warm water is comforting, like coffee, and it is also destressing and detoxifying. I love my warm water with lemon. Sometimes, I add honey too when I feel like something sweet."

Liza Huber's Mindless Moments

Susan's daughter and the *Passions* star Liza Huber loves to drive long distances to relax. She says, "I find it very therapeutic. I take Charlie, my golden retriever, listen to big band music like Harry Connick, Jr., and Frank Sinatra, and just drive for hours." Another mindless method of de-stressing for Liza is watching reruns of *The Golden Girls*. She explains, "It is a huge idiosyncratic love of mine. It is just such a funny show. When I am in a bad mood, I just turn on the reruns!" Liza also likes to write in her journal before going to sleep. As she explains it, "Writing helps to drain everything out of my head and allows me to get to bed."

Chapter Fourteen

Motivation Mantras

NOW THAT we have introduced you to so many serenity-boosting "me-time" possibilities, and, we hope, even inspired you to finally do something for yourself, it is time to implement the changes! We do understand that sometimes it takes more than a little nudge from a book to get you motivated enough to take action. Of course, you know that you should treat yourself to a massage, an indulgent bath, or some aromatherapeutic chocolate chip cookies, but for some odd reason you just can't seem to find a few moments to pull yourself away from your work, kids, and social life. Not to worry, we understand your pain and are sometimes guilty of the exact same thing. So we have asked a few of our gurus and celebrities to give us a bit of advice on how they get motivated.

Setting an Intention

The fitness trainer Gregory Joujon-Roche focuses much of his energy on discovering what sparks the interests of his clients through a process of self-awareness. A great way to begin this process, says Gregory, is through determining your intention. Similar to a goal, intention is the clarification of your purpose.

Gregory's Recipe for Setting a Fitness Intention

Ultimately, ask yourself, Why are you working out?

What do you wish to achieve? You may have a "superintention," say, to lose weight or be more flexible, maybe even both. You may have smaller, per workout intentions that support your superintention.

The clearer you are about your goal or intention, the easier it is to be aware during your workout and know whether you are succeeding and evolving.

Self-Monitoring

Another way to enhance clarity about your intention and monitor your progress is to write it down. Yep, journal it! Keeping a journal may sound cumbersome and impractical, but it has been shown to help motivate in a way similar to having a personal trainer. Journaling forces you to check in on yourself. Just keep it simple! Grab a calendar and simply write down what you did for yourself today and how it made you feel. If writing down your feelings is too involved, then grade them on a scale from 1 to 10 or scribble a happy, sad, or thrilled face. Of course, you can be more thorough and dedicate an entire page to each "me-time" activity. Describe what you did, why you did it, who you did it with, how it made you feel, and how much time you spent on it. You don't have to dedicate yourself to this task for the rest of your life; just keep a journal for three weeks or so, and honestly record what you have done for yourself. You will begin to see a pattern—what works and what doesn't. If the whole idea of journaling turns you off, then try a motivation mantra.

Gregory's Motivation Mantras

YOU'RE NUMBER ONE

It is so important to set aside "me-time" for your training and in life. Your workout time is sacred, and taking that time will give you the patience, creativity, and productivity you need to get through your day no matter how busy it can be. How can you give to others if you don't give to yourself? Remember, you're number one.

CAUGHT IN A FUNK?

Don't be frustrated with yourself if you're having a bad day, low energy, or your mind is muddled. Chances are there's a reason. Maybe you need to take a break. Take a moment to honor how you feel, then get back in. Find the flow and go with it. Try checking into where your desire level is. Get in touch with why you are doing what you are doing. Keep in mind that many times a workout can get you out of a funk, give you new perspective, and reenergize your day!

GET BACK TO CENTER

First, be still. Clear your mind. As thoughts and outside ideas pop in, acknowledge them and allow them to pop back out. Get back to you—your current mental, physical, and emotional being. Where are you at today? Take inventory; note anything unusual or any area of discomfort. This takes practice. Notice when you're somewhere else, and bring your thoughts and awareness back to center. Remember, when in doubt, a nice big breath will always take you there.

PRESENT MOMENT AWARENESS

Pay attention, be present! To be aware is to be in touch, open, listening, and focused on creating the results you desire. Expectations can throw the whole process into disarray. Honor where you are, not where you want to be. Stay here, not there. Here gets you there!

BACK TO BREATH!

The more in touch you are with your breath, the more you will achieve. If your intention is clear and connects through your breath to your body, you will see results manifest very quickly. So many people tune out; you must dial in, connect to the body, and breathe.

INTENT

Trust the intuitive and seek a new ideal of self as you surrender to the process of becoming who you choose to be. Reclaim your body, eliminate doubt, and replace it with intention. Just breathe and listen. Ego, fear, and all the rest just help reinforce who we are not.

With a Little Help from a Friend

Kelly Rutherford's boyfriend often helps her muster "me-time" motivation. She says, "You almost have to schedule it in. Sometimes, if I have been in a bad mood, my boyfriend will say, 'Have you had any girl time lately?' It reminds me that, no, I haven't gotten a facial or done a yoga class in a while and I need to do it. My mom once told me to get a bunch of beauty magazines, make myself a cup of tea, and just relax and read them."

Lauren Holly's best friend bullied her into relaxing. It may sound strange, but for some type A personalities, that's the only way to relax. Lauren recounts, "My best friend would always tell me to relax and sit down. I am definitely a type A personality; I mean, I have to have every dish in my sink cleaned before I can go to bed, and having someone force me into sitting down helped me finally to do it. When I sat, I realized how good it felt!"

The art guru Ed Buttwinick's students help to keep him motivated. "My students motivate me," he states. Conversely, a good teacher—one who is dedicated, caring, and can critique in a healthy way—is essential to a positive art experience. Ed advises, "Seek someone who can help you—a mentor, a class, even a book—for sustained motivation."

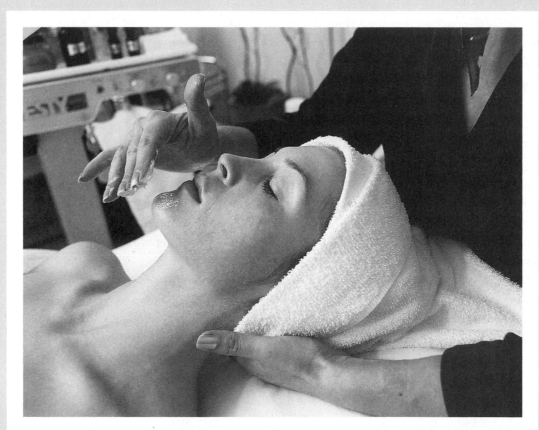

Kelly Rutherford being pampered.

A Gift of Motivation

Many of us have a passionate desire to do, create, or release, yet for some reason, we restrict our creative outlets and go on with our day-to-day. Jenna von Oy always longed to paint. While her career as an actress is certainly creative, there is just something about the freedom that you feel when grabbing hold of a paintbrush. Her boyfriend was aware of Jenna's desire, and he became the catalyst to her artistic release. As a Valentine's Day gift, he gave her an easel and paints, inspiring Jenna to enroll in a painting class in order to get those creative juices flowing.

Inner Inspiration

Some people are able to muster enough self-motivation to inspire themselves to set aside regular "time for their self." Marla Maples is one of them. She explains, "I am very self-motivating. I believe in pushing myself to relax and destress in order to be the best and most patient mother that I can be. I enjoy being able to give love to people who need it." But in order to give to others, you have to feel whole within yourself. "Me-time" can provide that strength and stability. "The harder something is to commit to, the harder you have to push to obtain it and the more you will get out of it. Sometimes, it is hard to find time for yourself. But it is so essential." If you are having trouble gathering enough self-generating motivation to actually put your good intentions in motion, Marla suggests creating a support system or group of friends who will encourage you on your sacred journey. "Community and friends are great modes of motivation!"

The Gift of Giving

Asha Blake is constantly giving information as a television journalist. But she doesn't get reciprocation from her viewers. Giving gifts to loved ones motivates her to hand-tint photographs, her "me-time" activity of choice. "When I do my hand-tinting projects for other people," she explains, "it's the joy on their faces that motivates me. Just to see how happy they are when they get a picture they don't expect is enough to keep me going."

A Family Affair

The celebrity personal trainer Gunnar Peterson's motivation to work out (his "me-time" activity) is his family. He says, "Your family is everything. It is your core. You want to be able to keep up with your kids." The fact is that one day the son will beat his dad in a one-on-one basketball game and the daughter will outrace her mom in a swimming contest; but don't you want to be in good enough shape at least to take your kids on?

If you don't have kids, Gunnar believes you have to work out in order to make good on your dreams. "If you have always wanted to travel to a tropical island, and you worked hard your entire life in order to make enough money to splurge and take that vacation, but once you get to the beach you are too ashamed of your bulging stomach and flabby thighs to get in a bathing suit, you will regret every lazy, exerciseless day that you wasted." So maybe a beach paradise is not your dream vacation but instead a trip to a faraway country. Imagine being a hundred pounds overweight, with weak knees and stiff joints. How is that fourteen-hour flight going to feel? Then, when you finally land, do you actually expect to be able to go on hours of walking tours without gasping for air? Take the time to take care of yourself, and you will have the opportunity to reap the rewards in the end.

As coauthor of this book (Sharon), I have come to analyze my own methods of "me-time" as well as what motivates me to carve out a few minutes a day for me. My daughters are my biggest motivators. They know that I am constantly trying to reclaim my past interest in drawing and painting. To keep me focused, my girls are always buying me art supplies and books about painting while insisting that we go to galleries. Last year my Christmas present from my youngest daughter, Julia, was a complete watercolor kit—paper, paints, brushes, and even a dish. She knew that if just one essential item were missing, I would have an excuse not to tackle the project. And I have really enjoyed sitting on my porch and painting the pots of flowers that line my patio. A couple of years ago, Laurel, my oldest daughter, gave me books on tile and mosaics, with a box of tiles and glue.

You would think that a commitment to fitness would come easy to the Kaehler-Koch household. However, even the fitness expert Kathy Kaehler uses some not so subtle fitness messages for her family. Her Hidden Hills gym may be home to A-list celebrities, however it is also the place where her husband and three young sons spend quality workout time. In order to keep them motivated, Kathy has tacked a gigantic paper workout schedule to the wall of the gym entitled "Koch Family Fitness." The chart gives the family a running tally of everyone's fitness accomplishments, by date, exercise, and repetitions. The exercises, including leapfrogging across the lawn and shooting five baskets, are fun and kid oriented. Each day has

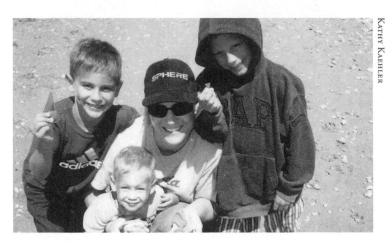

KATHY KAEHLER

Kathy Kaehler with her sons.

a requirement, and at the end of the week, the results are tallied. Kathy says, "The kids love seeing their progress—which spaces remain blank and which ones are filled. They particularly like challenging my husband and me. Friendly competition with parents is very motivating. And they love the reward at the end of the week, such as being treated to something that they really want to do or somewhere they want to go, without a sibling!"

Janet Gunn, actress, jewelry designer, and mother of a young son, is the consummate multitasker. For her, sleeping is more than a restful respite to a hectic schedule; it also provides the motivation for her jewelry designing. She says, "My motivation comes from the [jewelry] images I see in my sleep, which are hard to ignore. When I wake up, I am more motivated to create what I saw in my dreams!"

The actress Lisa Rinna finds "me-time" essential to her survival. She explains, "I need time for myself to survive! I also need it so that I can be there for my kids and my husband, my store and my acting job. If I don't take time off, no one gets the best of me."

To Your Health

I (Laurel) personally love "me-time," which is one of the reasons that I decided to co-write this book. Unfortunately, like many of you, I seem to forget just how essential my personal time is. In times of stress, when work and life in general are overwhelming—when, by the way, it would most behoove me to take a few moments for myself—I somehow neglect my "me-time." It's funny that while I was in the throes of writing this book, my friends would say, "Laurel, aren't you writing a book about destressing?" And then they would laugh, because I am one of the more stressed-out, high-strung women I know.

The problem is that when I forget to work out or take that five minutes a day simply to breathe, I get sick. It is as though my body is saying to me, "You don't want to slow down? You don't want to take care of yourself? Fine, then I will force you to." Suddenly, I have come down with a terrible cold or flu and I am restricted to the couch for days on end, feeling absolutely worthless, yet simultaneously masochistically loving every lazy moment. There you have it; I have to have "me-time" for the sake of my health. Plus, few people like to be in close proximity or even a phone call away from me when I am in a grouchy and overextended mood. So, for the sake of yourself, your family, and your friends, please, please, please treat yourself to "me-time" every day!

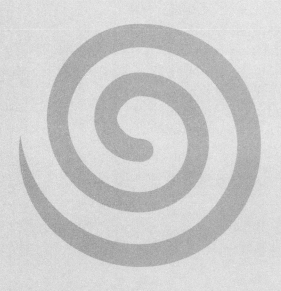

About the Authors

Laurel

Like many American women, I strive to have it all. In fact, I so badly wanted to be all grown up that, immediately upon graduating from college, I had my entire life mapped out—marriage at twenty-one, successful career by twenty-three, first child at twenty-five, and house by twenty-eight. Without a hitch, I rushed into a marriage with my college sweetheart at the ripe old age of twenty-one! Unfortunately, as was expected by everyone but me, that shotgun wedding quickly crumbled. But I didn't let that deter me. I had my sights set on a "big-time" career, which soon proved emotionally exhausting. After several setbacks, I finally realized that, yes, I could map out my life to the T, but most likely my life would pave its own path. Finally, at twenty-five years old, I have found Chris, my wonderful and supporting husband, a daily exercise regimen, enough close friendships to ensure that there is always an available ear to listen and a shoulder to cry on, a wonderful relationship with my family, and a successful career as a magazine editor and a freelance writer for various men's and women's publications.

Born and raised in Los Angeles, I became quite familiar with the fast-paced life of a trendy, up-and-coming overachiever, a self-proclaimed "do-everything" woman. But then one day I stopped, freaked out, and realized that I was on the path to becoming my mother, a woman who is so busy taking care of everything and everyone else that she often neglects to take care of herself. It was this sudden self-realization that lead to the concept of "me-time" and the focus of *The Gurus' Guide to Serenity.* Now I spend my days researching and writing about the little things in life that make people happy. From fitness and spas to gardening and cooking, I am here trying to save my own serenity as I teach others how absolutely essential it is to savor your "me-time," even if just for a few minutes a day.

Sharon

My last child is seventeen and tied up in her own world of schoolwork and friends. Although I should have time on my hands, I still can't seem to carve out space for myself. And many of my friends are "empty nesters" who have spent so little time on themselves that either they won't allow themselves to have some "me-time" or they don't know how to begin. I have seen many of my "stay-at-home" mom friends become paralyzed with fear as their last child goes off to college.

As a publicist with more than twenty years' experience, working with fitness and lifestyle gurus such as Richard Giorla of Cardio Barre, Gregory Joujon-Roche of Holistic Fitness, Gurmukh, the *Today* show's fitness expert Kathy Kaehler, and Jane Fonda's exercise line, I seem to be the one my friends call on when they want to know the latest stress-reducing exercise, relaxing facial, or creativity-boosting art class.

After talking to our guru clients, some of their celebrity clientele, magazine editors, and our friends, we decided to create a menu, with simple recipes for carving out time for yourself. The areas that we selected—baths and facials, massage, yoga and meditation, cooking, gardening, arts and crafts, sacred spaces, and exercise—are by no means the only solace-inducing remedies, however they were most mentioned by both the gurus and their celebrity clients with whom we spoke.